Biophotonics and Healing

By Steve Preston

2nd Edition 2018

Table of Contents

Introduction

This is an expanded version of the first edition of this book. Some of you may be wondering just what Bio-photonics is and what photo-Genetics has become. It is the study of electro-magnetic [E-M] emission or use of same in a biologic. This covers animals, plants, bacteria, and single cell elements of animals and plants. The major area of expansion in this edition is the expansion of the wavelengths investigated. This is not just about electro-magnetic waves we can see, but waves that extend from very low frequencies to the ultraviolet range of E-M photonic description. As you would expect, this book coves direct photonic ingress to change something about a biologic entity or promote healing. This healing extends from emotional stress, to cancer eradication. The book also is about the manufacture of and transmission of photonic and even low frequency E-M messages to communication or control other cells or entities outside the body or to remote organs of the body. The heart, for instance radiates far more E-M emissions than the brain and can still operate after direct connections with the brain are severed such a after heart transplant surgery. I think you will be amazed at what your own cells do and what plants do. Attempts to harness, control, use and adapt bio-photonic emissions is a very important advancement in our society but some harnessed this element of life long ago we will look at both old and new details to gain perspective needed.

A long time ago people began to realize that light played a role in living, but they had no idea just how important it would become.

- Three thousand years ago and before, some people would begin to glow as if the body generated bio-photonic bursts Some included the Biblical characters known as Angels, Jesus, Moses, and Noah. These emissions initiated fear. It would later be recognized these emanations occur in all of us to some degree.

- Two thousand years ago, the disciples of Jesus could heal sick by having contact with the skin of patients. Later we would learn that Bio-photonic message transfer from close proximity of individuals could, somehow, cure illnesses on occasion.

- In the 1600s Isaac Newton found that light could be split into its many colors by passing it through a prism. This started a massive search for what light was and what photons were. Even today we are not sure.

- Photo-Genetics is generally how scientists are able to control the brain with photo emissions.

-

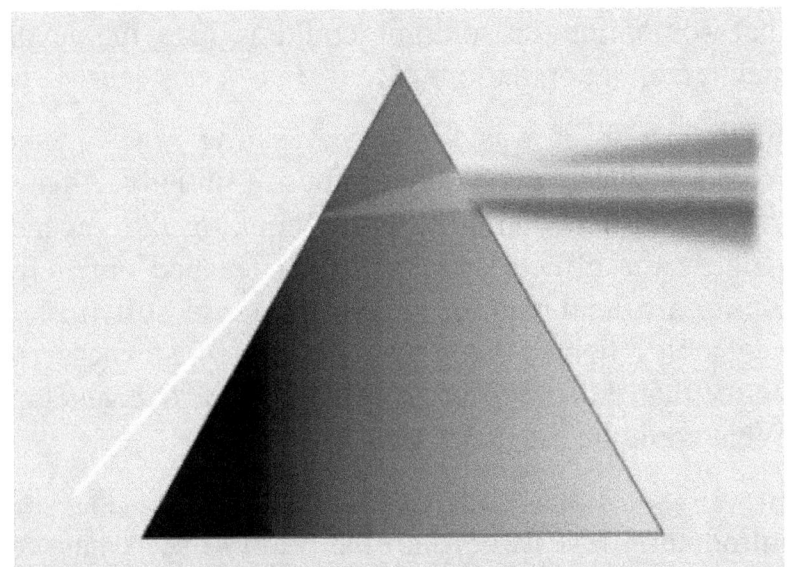

- In the 1700s it was determined that plants ingested light from the sun to increase strength and enhance growth. Photosynthesis investigators wondered what would happen if an animal got in the sunlight.

- Possibly as part of this investigation, someone would stay too long at the beach and the skin would burn. If they reduced the time, the skin would turn brown as the melanin in each cell would become activated to protect the skin and the rest of the body.

- Later they would find out that UV light would cause strange things to happen in skin cells. Sometimes cancer would form from the light.

- Some noted that people got sicker in the winter time when people did not go outside as often. Initially thinking it was the cold weather, soon it was determined that something in sunlight could <u>reduce the level of sickness</u> in a population.

- In the 1920s it was found that eating raw vegetables would reduce levels of sickness. Initially, this was thought to be vitamin based as cooking the vegetables reduces the effect as the vitamins leached out. After a while, artificial vitamins were tried and still fresh raw vegetables helped keep people free of sickness much better than all the vitamin pills and cooked vegetables. What could be the difference?

- In 1938, electroconvulsive therapy (ECT) started introducing EM waves into the brain to see what would happen. At first it was not well understood and cause damage, but later it was found to help the brain cells work better with an 86 percent remission rate for those with severe major depression.

- In the 1950s it was determined that sick plants could transmit warnings to other plants nearby to protect themselves. Initially, it was thought that Pheromone smells were sent out. It was discovered that the messages were ultraviolet optical messages.

- In the 60s apparent discharged electromagnetic waves were seen on photographic sheets. Called Kulian photography; live things, plant or animal, appeared to have sort of a halo. Even after death, the halo continued, but would dissipate.

- In 1970 it was found that cancer causing hydrocarbons would change UV light that these hydrocarbons would sense, while normal cells could retransmitted the same light. It was determined that limiting the UV light would slow the progressing of cancer.

- By 1972 a massive investigation on how the brain could be manipulated with extremely low frequency E-M waves provided shocking details and some were very curative. The problem was methods to emit these low frequencies to talk to the brain. An unsupported report indicated a sphincter relaxation frequency was found to be about 4 Hz. It was notoriously described as the "Brown Note".

- In the 1980s scientists found that blasting a cell with 380nm UV light such that 99 per cent of the cell, including its DNA, was destroyed could be completely reversed in a single day with very low doses of the same 380nm.

- In 1985 in an attempt to transmit extremely low frequency E-M waves into the brain to treat depressive issues, the Repetitive transcranial magnetic stimulation (rTMS) was developed, became an accepted treatment in the mid-1990s, and approved by the FDA in 2008. By increasing the frequency, this therapy also is treating seizure disorders.

- In the 1990 Bio-Photonic healing was noted as RED light would aid in all types of healing.

- In the 1990s John Hutchison was making matter disappear, become weightless and pass through objects using various E-M waves.

- By 1995 it was discovered that a mass of nerves in the Heart acted like a secondary brain. The interesting part wasn't understood until about 2004 when it was understood the heart brain actually could radiate farther than the head brain and could think on its own.

- In the 1990s we find a scientist that began discovering unbelievable things would happen if a body was irradiated by low frequency infrareds and high frequency microwaves. Some of the changes included invisibility and weightlessness. So far only inanimate objects have been used for subjects. Luckily, our atmosphere does not allow these signals to be radiated very far.

- Even with people emitting visible haloes of light 3 thousand years ago, it was not until about 2000 that experiments confirmed the skin and every cell in animals and plants emitted light called Bio-photons. When stressed, it was found there were more emissions in the stressed area so doctors could find cancer and disease locations easier.

- By 2010 all types of bio-photonic treatments for hair loss, recovery of circulation for diabetes, healing of wounds, reduction of pain, reduction in depression, reduced arthritis suffering, and many other things began to become popular.

- By 2011 Transcranial magnetic field treatments were extended to Rat studies testing reanimation of nerves in animals and enhanced fear extinction for Traumatic Stress Disorder and paralysis issues.

- By 2012 discovery of a complex optical coded messaging in plants and animals assured us of the great importance of bio-photonic emissions and detection.

- By 2013 Cancer was cured with Mistletoe optical messaging. While some insisted this was why people would kiss under the plant, but the kissing seems to have nothing to do with healing.

- In 2015 it was reported that UV messages from frog DNA were transmitted to salamander DNA and a frog was produced. These messages could increase growth or kill adjacent cells and adjacent entities.

To talk about this subject we will look at a number of sciences, investigations, experiments, treatments and outcomes along the lines of bio-stimulation and processes associated with bi-photonics as generally outlined below.

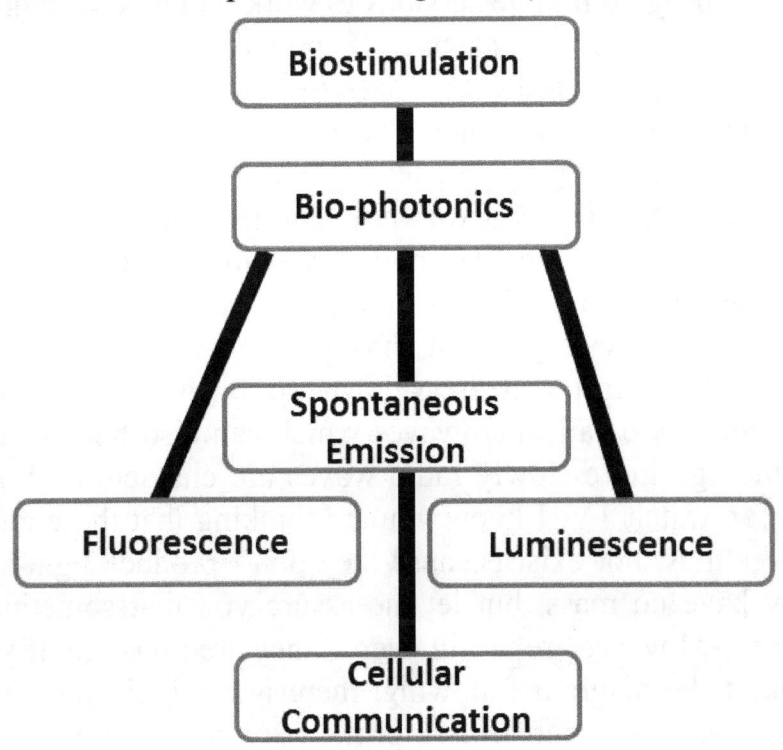

We are going to review all of these elements. I think we should find out what is happening inside our bodies so we can fix things.0. This book is to bring bio-photonics out of the snake oil salesman group and into more science so people will understand what is happening, have information that could help them use bio-photonics, and insure this important part of our anatomy is not disregarded.

Unfortunately, the Chakra controllers and Acupuncture quasi-doctors are making it somewhat difficult. I don't know that the way I presented the details will be much better, but I assure you I'm not trying to sell a bio-photonic treatment machine that sparkles and flashes and changes color during 90 minute sessions to work on mood changing. I am looking for real change. To initiate these changes we will look at a wide variation in Photonic or Electro-Magnetic wave frequency. There is an electromagnetic wave or frequency associated with the color of the light [Whatever that is!], but we know that the faster the photon of light thing vibrates the more powerful it becomes. Soon the fast vibrating photon thing becomes dangerous to humans as it can go right through the body [x-ray]. We won't go that fast. If it slows down too much it changes into something we call microwaves which can also hurt us, but as they go more slowly radio waves are characterized and we can watch TV. I know you are thinking that these radio waves must not exist because they don't produce light and they have no mass, but let me assure you that sometimes these E-M waves are useful even if they are invisible. If you look at the diagram following, there is a wiggly line. The faster wiggling represents a prime particle vibrating faster and faster. Radio waves are sensed as light that finally turns into the deadly gamma rays. For this book we need all frequencies from Ultra-violet to almost no vibration at all.

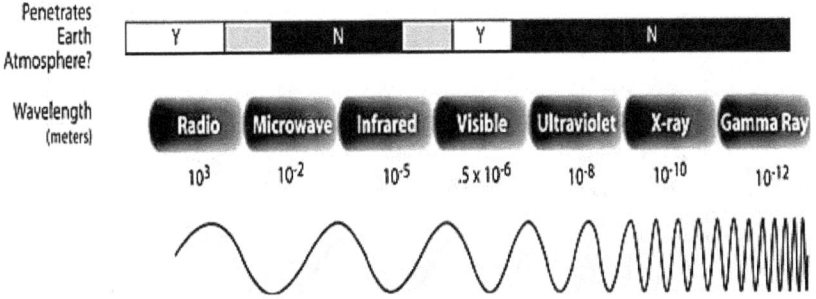

- **Ultraviolets** excite DNA directly and seem to be the main retransmission wavelength of cells.
- **Visible Wavelengths** can be absorbed through the skin.
- **Infrared**- In some cases Infrareds absorb more deeply than visible wavelengths.
- **Microwaves** seem to change the structure of material so there is substantial interest in its curative powers.
- **Radio waves** are interesting to listen too.
- **Subsonic E-M emissions**- Substantial work is being done at wavelengths well below those we can hear. Manufacturing them is the trick.

This book deals with emissions <u>into</u> the body to support testing, modification and curative possibilities as we as the emissions <u>from</u> the body that do similar things. One interesting emitting organ of the body, the heart, is a fairly new focal point for studies as its 40 thousand neuron, E-M Field radiating brain has changed the concept and curative possibilities studied in recent years.

Bio Photons

As I briefly introduced, it has been known for some time now that our body, all other animals, and all plants transmit, receive, and interpret photonic messages. Depending on how they are sent, things change in nearby cells or even nearby people or plants. While the majority of the emissions are in the Ultraviolet range, some are visible. The levels are low as the photon communications are for short distances.

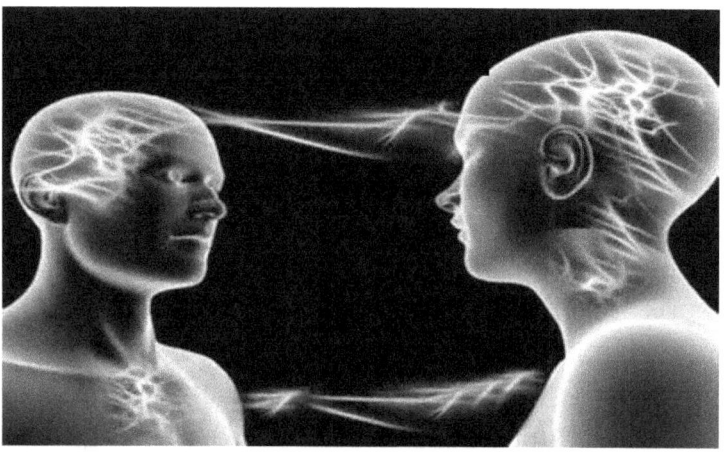

The image above might show how feelings and image transfers might look if we could see them. I think the best example is when someone cuts their hand open. The body needs to repair itself, so the affected cells send out a distress photonic message to the nearby "good" cells" that they need to replicate. The cells get that message, replicate, and, soon the cut is completely gone. Please notice the emissions from the Heart. We will look at that later. The messages are by pulse coding and differences in output wavelength. The most complicated and manipulative higher frequency bio-photonic generators and receivers are in the molecules known as DNA while extremely low frequencies are transferred by the neuron clusters in the head and heart.

DNA Emits, Detects, and Decodes Visible and UV Photons

One of the leaders in this study of light is a Russian scientist named Pjotr Garjajev. He recently was able to intercept UV Photonic communication from a DNA molecule from one organism, a frog embryo, and retransmit it to another organism's DNA, a salamander embryo, causing the latter embryo to develop into a frog! Evidently what happens is the DNA sends out a message that can be seen by cells passing nearby, if they receive a particular optical message, they might turn into skin, or whatever. The main thing is that the old idea that everything was accomplished by chemical modifications making electrical differences that were interpreted by cells has now been thrown away. Light builds people, animals, and plants.

Plants Emit, Detect and Decode

A Russian biologist was the first to find this out. His name was Alexander Gurwitsch who experimented on onion cells and found that stimulating one onion that was near another would cause the second one to flourish if there was quartz between them but not if silicon was between them because the biophotons that were being transmitted were Ultra-violet. With no barrier or quartz, one onion being fed would cause another to react. That whole concept of talking to your plants is gone------ now you need to send the right photons and they need to be the UV light. After the Onion Tests, I figured hospitals were not the place to be if one was sick unless people were placed in separate rooms or something that would halt UV light separated sick people. Plants would call out to those nearby not with pheromones but with light. The image below shows a cry for help and insecticide is sprayed. The photonic emission shouts out the fear and hurt and soon settles down.

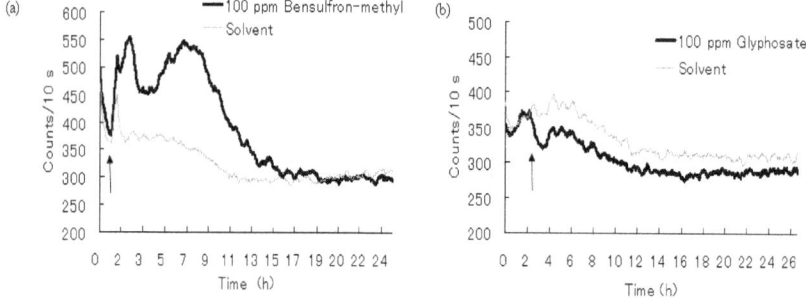

Photo-repair Sensing

Here is a strange thing! It seems that scientists found that blasting a cell with 380nm UV light so that 99 per cent of the cell, including its DNA, was destroyed was not the end of the cell. All you need to do is reblast the cell with a very low dose of 380nm and the cell will regenerate in a single day! I know that sounds like the rapid growth of cancer so let's see what happens there.

Hydrocarbons Detect and Emit

Some believe this Photo-repair messaging may be the cure for cancer. A theoretical biophysicist at the University of Marburg in Germany named Fritz-Albert Popp started his work in 1970, examining differences in a carcinogenic hydrocarbon named benzoapyrene, and almost identical but safe one named benzoepyrene. Again, UV light was the thing to activate photonic emission of these cells, He had illuminated both molecules with ultraviolet (UV) light in an attempt to find exactly what made these two almost identical molecules so different. The first one emitted a different frequency while the safe hydrocarbon reemitted the same frequency. He found out that other cancer-causing hydrocarbons did the same type of photon change and they would only react to 380 nm. Once activated Massive output of photons erupt from cancerous cells to invigorate those nearby as shown below.

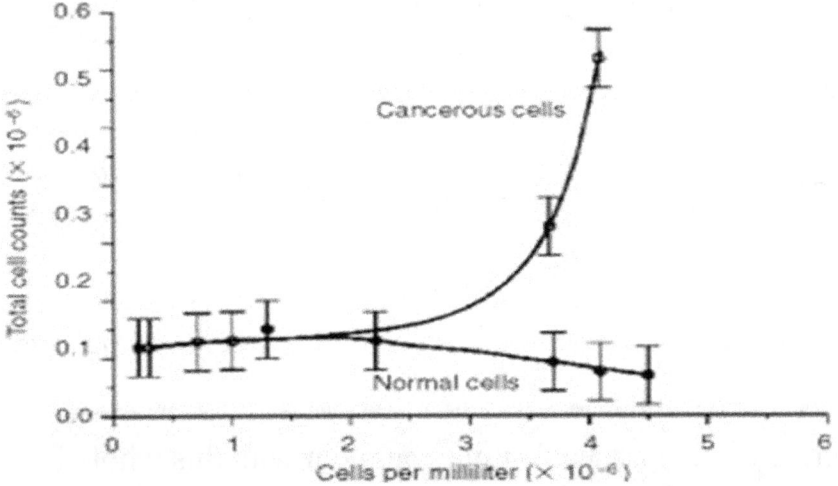

It was also noted that Melanin is capable of transforming ultraviolet light energy into heat such that more than 99.9% of the absorbed UV radiation is transformed from potentially genotoxic (DNA-damaging) ultraviolet light into harmless heat, but destruction of that safeguard would quickly allow 380nm signals to begin changing cells.

Photons Control Everything

It seems Photons switch on and control ALL the body's processes. Given different frequencies, identical cells perform different functions. The question that has forever puzzled cellular biologists for decades has been, *"What is it that enabled the tens of thousands of different kinds of molecules in the organism to recognize their specific targets?"* We now are beginning to understand how it is happening. It's not helping us define what photons are and what light is, but it is given us the details we need to begin to construct a definition.

God

In the very first part of the first chapter of the book of Genesis, we read the following:

In the beginning God created the heavens and the earth. Now the earth was formless and empty; darkness was over the surface of the deep. The Spirit of God was hovering over the waters. God said, "Let there be light," and there was light. God saw that the light was good. He separated the light from the darkness. The evening and the morning were the first day.

Here are some issues that may help out with this whole Bio-photonics stuff.

1. It says *"God created the Heavens"*, but he didn't create the sun, moon, and stars yet, so there is question about what the heavens were.

2. The word *"NOW"* shows that the earth and heavens originally had form, but lost it.

3. *Darkness was over the surface of the deep* is also strange in that God had not made the sea yet. All of a sudden *God was hovering over the waters* when there was not sea.

4. This making of *"light"* was "four days" or 4-periods before he created the Sun, stars, and moon, that would eventually produce light, so the light created in this section came from something else.

5. Finally, God separated this "light" from the *"Darkness of the deep"*.

If we read the next part it even gets weirder, but I think this is all we need for now.

To read this little section one must understand a few things.

- The Hebrew word *Yawm'* simply means "time period" rather than 24-hour type of day. When the Bible says "day of famine" it doesn't mean the famine only lasted a 24-hour period. Besides there was no sun or moon yet.

- The word waters/*Mayim* actually means "life giving juice or simply life-giving place as water could give life". If the word was to be regular water it would have been *Ahava*, which means "regular water".

- The word Darkness/*Chashekh* means misery or destruction type of darkness.

- The word deep/*Thom* means the abyss type of deep.

Given a more modern way of saying this section without changing the words, we can see the following is easier to understand.

*In the beginning God created the heavens and the earth. After a while, the earth was destroyed and so was the rest of the universe. Then God remade life He created the **"light of life"** and without this light there was death. This all happened during the first period of our world.*

The "light of life" described over 3 thousand years ago was what this book is about. Our entire body works on E-M field generation of coded messages that allow our cells to work as a single component. The coded messages can be generated by brain action or by cell receiving signals from damaged cells needing help. I'm not saying a cell has a brain, but to understand the electromagnetic emission of the body better, we must open out minds to new discoveries the major one we are addressing here is how the Heart initiates phot-communications both to other components of our body and to the outside world. To help you understand this new science, let me first redefine our being as a cognizant observer.

Triune Entity

To understand the photonic/E-M messaging more completely we must understand something called Heart-brain messaging, and we must recognize our complete self. We are cognizant of ourselves in the visible reality [by our Head-Brain], our concept of reality is sort-of controlled [by something called the soul], and communication outside our universe [by something called our spirit]. Scientists a now telling us without these levels of cognition, nothing would exist. We are finding out that we cannot interface with the soul or spirit part of us without the almost unbelievable capabilities of our heart. Yes; I said the heart and a number of scientists are giving us the first glimpses into this new direction for bio-science. Another way of showing our triune entity is next. The heart communicates with all three. For this book I will be talking about an important link between separate dimensions of our being as the heart does a lot more than pump blood.

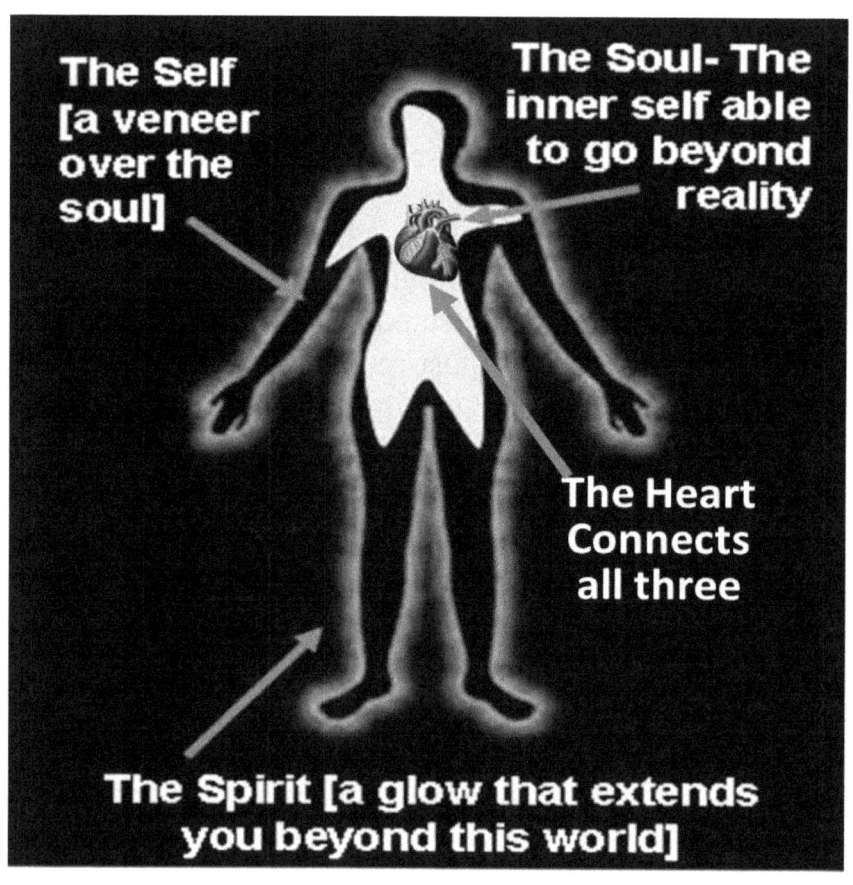

The Self [a veneer over the soul]

The Soul- The inner self able to go beyond reality

The Heart Connects all three

The Spirit [a glow that extends you beyond this world]

As we dig into the capabilities of the Heart and its Photonic messaging, we will have to look beyond our "self" portion a little, so some of this may sound a little bizarre if you have not had instruction on the three entities of our being, so I will try to expand your awareness as slowly as I can. First let's look for verification in an unlikely location. The next graphic provides a general accounting of how the Heart provides this messaging between our separate beings.

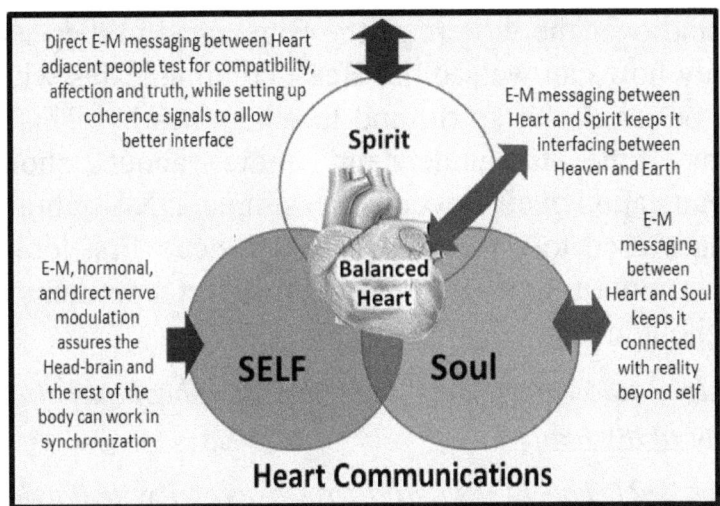

Heart Communications

Some details can be provided in the Bible, but it is different than you may have been taught in church. First of all, the heart is not the seat of compassion as you have been told. That was introduced to you because we really had no knowledge of what the heart really was. It is easy to see that the center of compassion was the bowels for the Early Egyptians and the Jews writing the Bible and shown in the next verses.

*I John 3:17-But whoso hath this world's good, and seeth his brother have need, and shutteth up his **bowels of compassion** from him, how dwelleth the love of God in him?*

*Colossians 3:12-Put on therefore, as the elect of God, holy and beloved, **bowels of compassion**, kindness, humbleness of mind, meekness, long-suffering;*

Now for the meat. Almost every single book of the Bible describes elements of our heart we try our best to ignore.

Over and over the writers of the Bible tried to help us out, but only now can we see the Heart communicates with our brain, our soul, our spirit, and to others nearby. This is an exciting time to understand more about photonic-communication well beyond the simple DNA vibrational messages used to repair cells nearby. Let's first look at a tiny portion of the 150 verses on Heart communication throughout the Bible.

Genesis 24:45 *"Before I [servant of Abraham] finished* <u>*praying in my heart*</u>*---*

Exodus 4:21 *The LORD said to Moses, - I will* <u>*harden his [Pharaoh's] heart*</u>

Deuteronomy 4:29 <u>*seek the LORD your God with all your heart and with all your soul*</u>*.*

1 Samuel 17:28 *I [Eliab talking to David] know how conceited you are and* <u>*how wicked your heart is*</u>*; you came down only to watch the battle."*

1 Kings 3:9 *give your servant* <u>*a discerning heart*</u> <u>*to govern your people and to distinguish between right and wrong*</u>*.*

Jeremiah 9:26 *even the whole house of Israel is* <u>*uncircumcised in heart*</u>*."*

Psalm 64:6 *Surely the* <u>*human mind and heart are cunning*</u>*.*

Proverbs 6:25 <u>*Do not lust in your heart*</u> *after her beauty or let her captivate you with her eyes.*

2 Chronicles 32:26 *Hezekiah repented of the* <u>*pride of his heart*</u>*.*

Nehemiah 9:8 *You* <u>*found his heart faithful*</u> *to you.*

Ezekiel 25:6 <u>rejoicing with all the malice of your heart</u>

Isaiah 13:7 every <u>heart will melt with fear</u>.

Hosea 10:2 Their <u>heart is deceitful</u>,

Matthew 15:19 out of the <u>heart come evil thoughts—</u> <u>murder, adultery, sexual immorality, theft, false testimony,</u> <u>slander</u>

Mark 12:33 To <u>love him with all your heart</u>, with all your understanding and with all your strength,

Acts 2:26 <u>my heart is glad</u> and my tongue rejoices

Romans 9:2 Sorrow and unceasing <u>anguish in my heart</u>

1 Corinthians 4:5 He will expose the <u>motives of the heart</u>.

2 Corinthians 2:4 I wrote you out of <u>great distress and</u> <u>anguish of heart</u> and with many tears,

Ephesians 1:18 I pray that the <u>eyes of your heart may be</u> <u>enlightened.</u>

Colossians 3:22 Slaves, obey your earthly masters with <u>sincerity of heart</u>.

1 Timothy 1:5 love, which comes from <u>a pure heart</u> and a good conscience and a sincere faith. This is a very important verse in that it is talking about "true love" of someone besides "self". This can only be achieved by empowering the soul by means of a communicating heart.

Philemon 1:20 <u>Refresh my heart in Christ</u>.

Hebrews 3:12 None of you has <u>a sinful, unbelieving heart</u> that turns away from the living God.

Heart take a controlling function in many of the things you thought your head-brain did. With that as an introduction, let's look at Heart-brain bio-genetics

Heart Brain Biogenetics

I know all those descriptions sounded religious and spiritual and all that, but what we are finding out about the heart and its brain [a real separate brain inside your heart] are just about as "religious" as that presented in the Biblical testimony, but now it is being found and tested in a laboratory. The heart seems to be able to do all of this stuff. Scientists have now found that the heart is more than just a pretty face. It has its own 'stand alone" brain, endocrine system, communication/sight, and control over our bodies and sometimes, even our head-brain. Instead of being a massive clump, like the head-brain, the neurons of the heart-brain are localized throughout the main vessels of the pump part and the various sections are all interconnected.

- 20% of these neurons have to do with mechanical information (pressure etc)

- The other 80% are sensitive to chemical substances (hormones, neurotransmitters) and set up actions that can allow the Heart to see and communicate.

I know that sounds like we ran out of brain, but we will see the Heart-brain is way more mysterious. This information gathers in the little brain in the heart, where it is integrated and used for local decision making. The Intrinsic neuro-system of the heart is also directly connected with skin, lungs and other organs so the Heart can control these body parts much faster than the head-brain using photon/E-M messaging.

While the Heart has a brain, it is a tiny thing by any definition so having all the previously described capabilities seems improbable when compared to the head –brain that is massive. The Heart brain elements are made up of about 40 thousand neurons while the head-brain is made up of something like 18 billion. While we are told no one uses more than 10% of our brain, we actually use much, much less than that and substantial amounts of our head-brain are bogged down in interpreting E-M signals that are turned into chemical charges by the sight sensor eyes. The brain takes the mesh of varied E-M signals and creates vision. The head-brain also takes vibrating pressure signals that are turned into chemical charges and builds appropriate meaningful "sounds". The head-brain also establishes characteristic muscle contractions needed to support vibrating our vocal cords for voice modulation and even "singing" for some of us.

Head-Brain Freedom

Generally speaking, the Heart-brain doesn't need to do any of that. If it needs that information, the Head-brain can get it like going to a library or the internet or using a calculator rather than trying to do math, so maybe, 40 thousand neurons not required to do the daily bookkeeping chores is enough to accomplish some remarkable effects. While we might thing of the Head brain as this master memory of carnal events, saying, songs, etc, the Heart-brain could be thought of as the glue that holds the three portions of your entity together. Separate the Soul, Spirit, and Self are not alive, so in a way, the Heart-brain allows us to be alive.

Neuroscientists today tell us the heart and its brain are far more complex than we'd ever imagined. Instead of simply pumping blood, it may actually direct and align many systems in the body so that they can function in harmony with one another. To make this seem even more surreal, this new scientific evidence shows that the heart uses various methods <u>to send our brain extensive emotional and intuitive signals and it does the same to heart-brains of other people nearby and it may even affect the reality of the world itself.</u> The heart is in constant communication with the brain and scientists are now beginning to believe that our hearts are the "intelligent force" behind the intuitive thoughts and feelings we all experience. Location of the Brain Ganglia that make up the heart-brain as shown in the heart cross-section below.

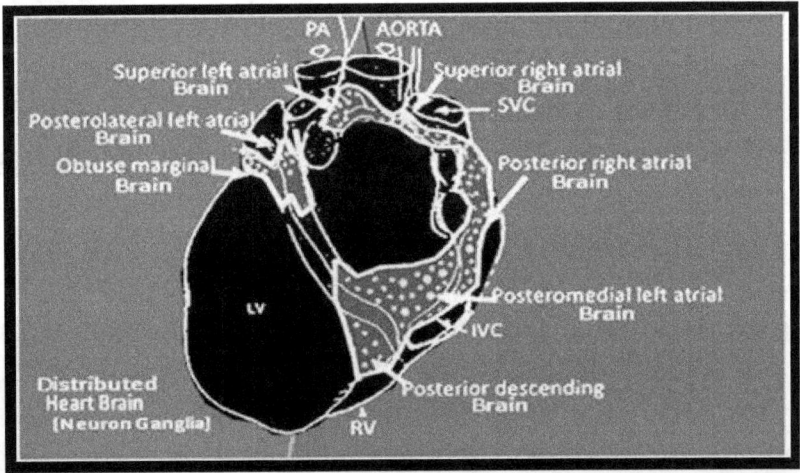

The way the heart communicates is remarkable. Not only can the heart recognize itself as an entity, it can modify Hormones to initiate E-M messaging and it can send frequency modulated messages alone the bloodstream to all parts of the body to communicate as shown next. Notice how your blood is not pumped at any one specific rate. Instead it is modulated.

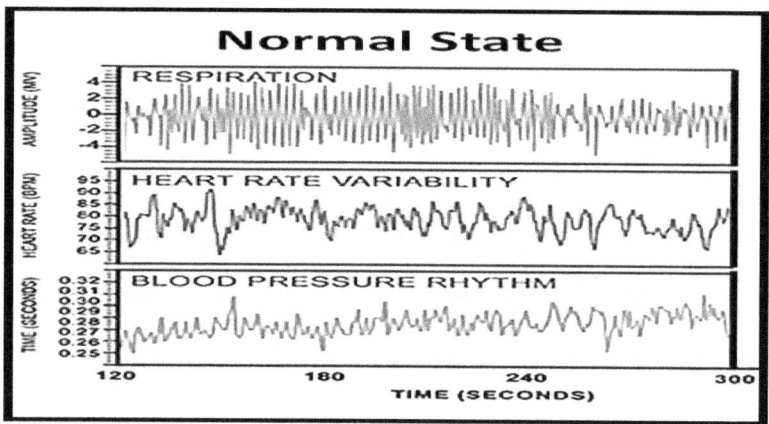

Some can focus the heart rhythms into a tight grouping of frequencies. When this happens, the heart not only can communicate with elements of the body, but <u>outside the body as well</u>. This is called Coherent communication. Coherent heart rhythm patterns are sent to the brain and the effect has been recorded. The effect is often experienced as <u>heightened mental clarity</u>, <u>improved decision making and increased creativity</u>. Additionally, coherent input from the heart tends to facilitate the experience of <u>positive feeling states</u>. This may explain why <u>most people associate love and other positive feelings</u> with the heart and why many people actually feel or sense these emotions in the area of the heart. As shown in the following graphic, if the Heart wants to communicate the pulse rate variations or spectrum is greatly reduced causing the Blood flow 'Power Spectral Density' (PSD) to spike as a higher power E-M event. With this focused electro-magnetic emission capability. The heart greatly extends what our head brain does and our DNA with respect to Photonic communication throughout the body and outside the body.

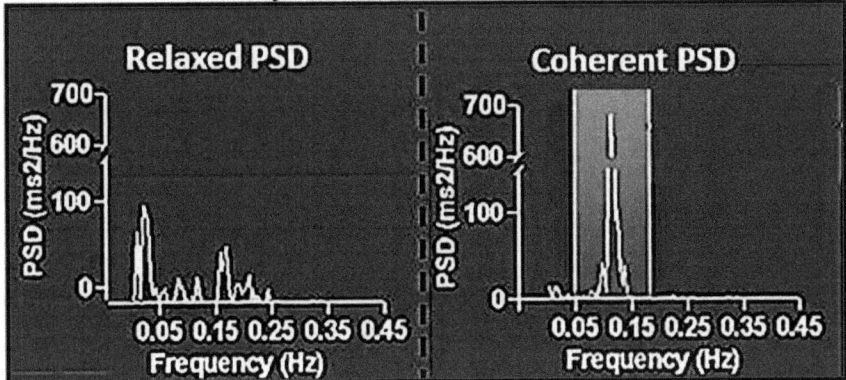

This whole heart-brain and its communication capabilities was established back in 1994 by Dr. Armour. His work revealed that the heart has a complex intrinsic nervous system that is sufficiently sophisticated to qualify as a 'brain' in its own right. His report indicated the following: *The heart's brain is an intricate network of several types of neurons, neurotransmitters, proteins and support cells similar to those found in the brain proper. Its elaborate circuitry enables it to act <u>independently</u> of the cranial brain – to learn, remember, and even feel and sense. Information from the heart; including feeling sensations, is sent to the brain through several pathways. These main nerve pathways enter the brain at the area of the medulla, and cascade up into the higher centers of the brain, where they may influence perception, decision making and other cognitive processes.*

It was later research by Dr. McCraty, in 2004, that was described this way. *The heart generates the body's most powerful and most extensive rhythmic electro-magnetic [Photonic] field. The heart's magnetic component is about*

500 times stronger than the brain's magnetic field and can be detected several feet away from the body. There is now evidence that a subtle yet influential electro-magnetic or 'photonic' communication system operates just below our conscious awareness. Energetic interactions possibly contribute to the 'magnetic' attractions or repulsions that occur between individuals, and also affect social relationships. It was also found that one person's brain waves can synchronize to another person's heart.

Research in the past two decades has shown that the heart is an information processing center that can learn, remember, and act independently of the cranial brain sending E-M messages. It seems we have a second "brain" in our chest and it is looks like Heart brains communicate with each other over their E-M/photonic communication channel. If we find out how to talk to it we may even cure lovesickness.

Now scientists are studying the "introspective awareness" of the heart itself, just like we learn from the 513 specific Bible verses, mostly describing a person's heart-communication and independence from our normal consciousness. So, we find three major Photonic/E-M communicators in our bodies. DNA focuses its communication to adjacent cells. The Head-Brain converts E-M messaging from our eyes as converts it to Light and sends messages to our guts to allow it to operate depending on E-M messaging from our various sensors. The heart-brain E-M communication not only modifies mood and love, but also can send messages outside out bodies to communicate with others, and initiate repair because of its huge emission director of sorts.

Heart-Brain E-M Emitter

When the heart brain is attuned by coherence, it can transmit outside the body with signal over 500 times as strong as that of the head brain and it is a very low frequency that modulates in mostly unidentified ways. Here is the thing to know if you want to successfully emit low frequency E-M signals; you MUST have a large emitter. One of the reasons for the Heart-brain's massive capability is the emitter itself. The Heart-brain used variations in blood flow using the entire body's blood vessel system to focus messaging as needed. Please notice the blood vessels produce and almost complete image of our bodies as shown next.

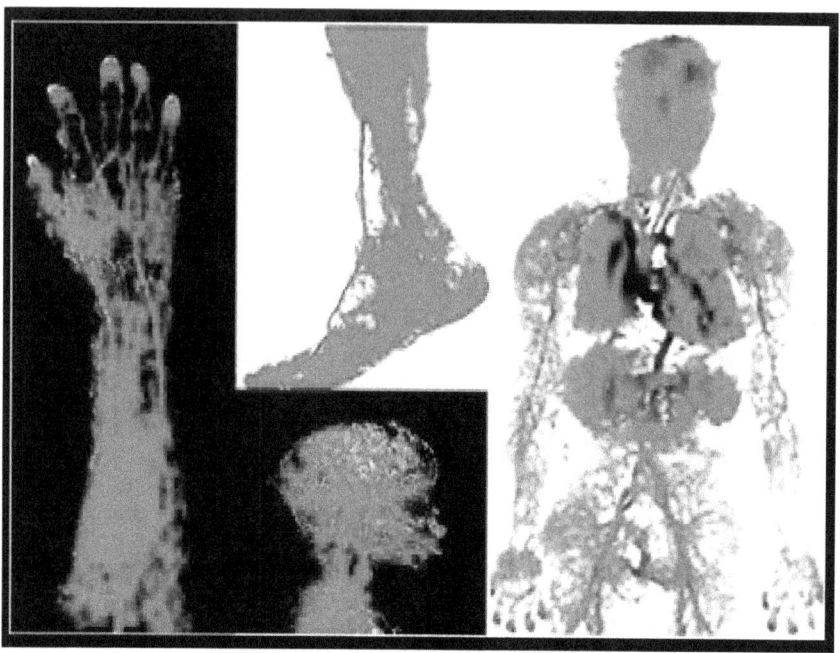

Each time there is a push of charges material it changes the magnetic field produced and when the pressure is released, another opposite phase E-M signal is produced and this emission is along the track of blood. While the head looks like a big pool of pulsating blood, the rest of the body is just about as dense as the whole body emits whatever the blood does. The images do not show the delicate capillary blood flow that just about fills in the rest of the images and we need to understand something about E-M emission here. They work off surface area so even the fine capillaries add to and generated field. Please notice something important. If you wanted to send messages to another heart-brain, one reasonable way would be to place hands on the other person as the fingertips are loaded with the high message content blood vessels. The Bible indicated that if we wanted to enhance healing possibilities, we should place our hands-on those needing healing or encouragement. This limited healing range is identified over and over again in the Bible as it continues to expand our awareness of our Heart-brain. I want you to notice something. I made a quick sketch showing a radar transmitter, TV receiver, and a faith healer placing his hands on someone. Do you see any similarities? If not, I'm sorry about my artwork. All the pulsing blood vessels pulse in unison and the signal is amplified by the sheer size of the emitter. Let's see what the Bible says again. By the way, the reason I am using the Biblical statements so much in this book is not for religion so much but because the Bible gives us a lot of information that is continuously being confirmed.

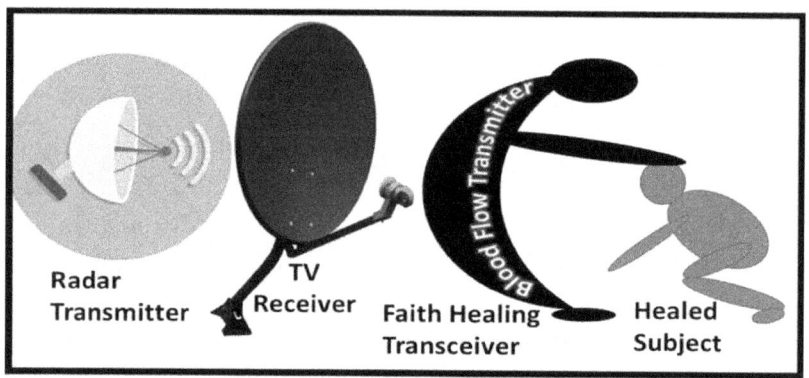

Radar Transmitter | TV Receiver | Faith Healing Transceiver | Healed Subject

How the heart communicates with the souls and spirit are not well understood, but let's look at the laying on of hands to heal the sick. Like just about everything else this uses E-M or Photonic message transmission. Our healing communication generally goes through our hands and we are told about this form of Photonic/E-M messaging over and over again.

The Biblical stories tell us that if we have "faith" we can heal by simply placing our hands on an injured person. But there might be more to this and the various faith healers that try to use hypnotheropy or grand utterances from a pulpit, or smashing someone on the head while in a state of trance, or building up one's CHI and sending something through a person's body to cure. All these "techniques" seem to have some success in treating a wide assortment of issues but sometimesa the "healing" is limited just like normal doctor's results using fancy herbs made in laboratories that had apparently helped a rat feel better. Let's see what these methods might really be doing.

Christian Laying on of Hands-Christian Laying on of hands is an extremely ancient method to cure disease of all types even up to death itself. The problem is it takes something called faith and the definition of that is somewhat obscure. Some thought it takes trust in God, but as I mentioned earlier, the faith described for faith healing is not the same as the Trust in God Faith needed for salvation. Therefore, many non-believers [and charlatan ministers] are still able to lay hands on people and cure them. The images below are of Catholic priests practicing it and a painting showing Jesus helping the sick.

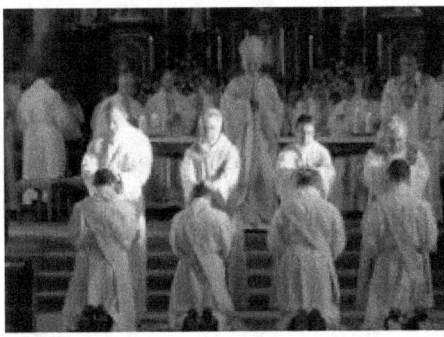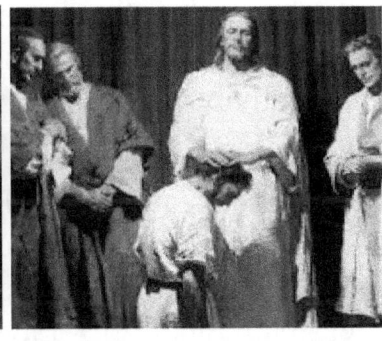

This faith stuff seems to work very well in this application so we had better learn about it. Laying hands on the sick was a common practice in the Early Church. Throughout the New testament we read over and over again about Jesus, his disciples and charlatan ministers laying their hands on patients and curing them. In Mark 16:18, Jesus said concerning His disciples, *"they will place their hands on sick people, and they will get well"*

This form of faith is simply an understanding and interconnection between self and the perceived reality we live in—sort of like the self-actualization of Abraham Maslow, but one step more intense. By "KNOWING" one can emit this "energy" and focusing on that event one can do it and people can be cured as the heart goes into a high level of coherency as described earlier. The Biblical stories tell us that if we have "faith" we can heal by simply placing our hands on an injured person. But there might be more to this and the various faith healers that try to use hypnotheropy or grand utterances from a pulpit, or smashing someone on the head while in a state of trance, or building up one's CHI and sending something through a person's body to cure. All these "techniques" seem to have some success in treating a wide assortment of issues. As most of the other "treatments" acocmplished in the normal medical world are failures, let's see what these methods might really be doing.

While I'm not getting into "faith" in this book as an act of honor to the creator God, all I want to say is that something called faith seems allow us to make our body photonic messaging coherent and more powerful to work so we had better learn about it. Laying hands on the sick was a common practice in the Early Church. Jesus often laid hands on people before healing them as described in Mark 6:5; Luke 4:40; and Luke 13:13. Jesus was somewhat different than normal men, but Paul laid hands on a sick person and he was healed in Acts 28:8.

So, Peter and at least 84 others cured many using only their hands with some communicative emanations from them about 2000 years ago.

As far I as can tell, the description of faith concerning healing of sick and doing a number of miraculous things had nothing to do with the "loving God faith", it simply was an understanding and interconnection between self and the perceived reality we live in—sort of like the self-actualization of Thomas Maslow, but one step more intense. By KNOWING one can emit this "energy" one can do it and people can be cured. This is similar to Somatic Therapy in the general sense but one would just heal himself to perform this action.

Somatic Therapy-The discovery of bio-photon emission and photonic messaging lends scientific support to some unconventional methods of healing based on concepts of self-regulation of the organism, or homeostasis. One such technique is called somatic therapy. The word somatic is derived from the Greek word "soma" which simply means living body. Somatic therapy is a holistic therapy that studies the relationship between the mind and body in regard to psychological past.

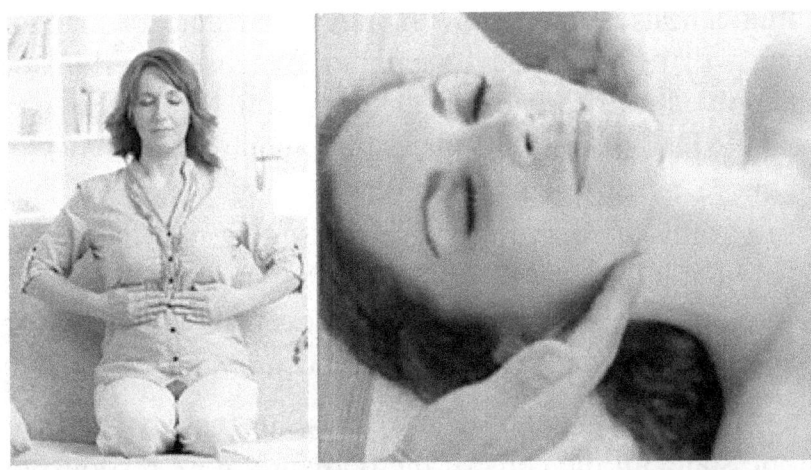

The images above show typical pressure initiated for Somatic Therapy. The theory behind somatic therapy is that trauma symptoms are the effects of instability of the autonomic nervous system [ANS]. Past traumas disrupt the ANS, so applying pressure at certain areas of the body or changing posture is said to remove these traumas. I don't know about all that, but if you change the shape of cells by pressure or posture, you could, very well, change the retransmission of various frequencies of light throughout your body. If restrictions of flow of bio-photonic emissions are caused by nerve cells not having the right fluids to produce or retransmit the right colors, this will change how we feel, how our cells operate, and a wide assortment of sicknesses and ailments will be assured. There is no doubt that something is going on, and we are slowly beginning to understand just what is making some people feel better by a simple touch.

Let's think about these nerves just a bit. When electrons move between energy states during chemical reactions as part of metabolic processes and as part of the cell to cell communication associated with nerve cell data exchange, photons will be absorbed or emitted. We used to think it was simply the difference in electron volt levels between nerve cells that allowed for messaging, but now we have so much more as different color photons are generated and affect not only the nerve to nerve messaging, but the entire body around the nerves. In Hypnotherapy, the "Healer" adds another level by increasing the level of suggestion of the patient, but the same method still occurs.

Hypnotherapy-In hypnotherapy, it is suggested that in a hypnotic state, all the cells of the body are more responsive to suggestions of healing. We can see from the hypnotherapy session shown next that the hands are placed very close or on the body at different times, even if the "patient" is not looking at them. This has nothing to do with hypnotism, it's something else. With the right lighting, there seems to be light coming from his hands.

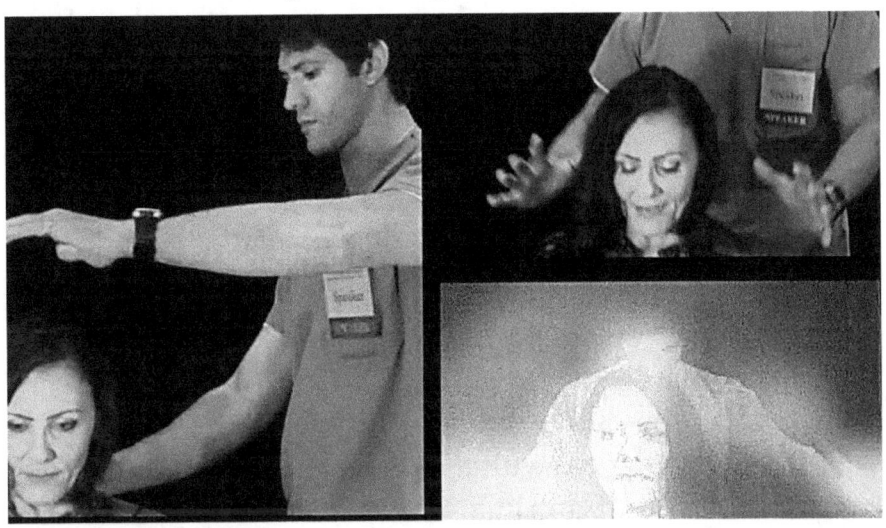

Chi Treatments-Chi treatments are a little different in that instead of allowing easier healing from relaxation, the healer uses a strong "faith" in his training. Very few peopkle have gotten this CHI which essentially is a focused energy in the body. By meditation, diet, and some other secret things, masters of Chi can, somehow, heal people by directing this internal energy into a wound or disorder to modify it.

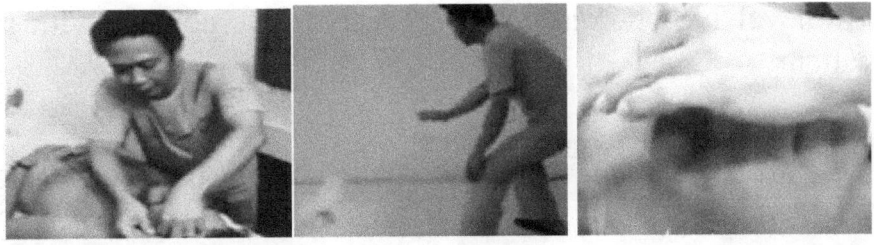

A demonstration of energy focus is shown above with extended accupuncture treatments, making flames appear and simply touching someone to cure issues. This is no joke. It seems to work, but hopefully, you see the hands on the person is, again a real part of this treatment. The focusing of energy may also give us a clue that large amounts of electrically induced photonic emissions are forced into a person so cells can be redirected. The "prana" of Indian Yoga physiology, apparently, is similar to this Chi energy concentration and their hands can heal as well.

Body Psychotherapy-Just like treating disease, laying on of hands seems to work for depression and other psychological disorders. You might see a body psychotherapist if you've got a persistent case of the blues; to help you cope during a troubled time, such as a death in your family; or to deal with the effects of a past trauma, like being the victim of a crime. The patient simply lies down while a therapist touches different spots on the body. In one account a therapist simply touched the back of the neck of a patient and it triggered a terrifying memory. Through the hands touching as the memory is realized, it is lessened. It is like having a psychologist with fingers.

Let me give you a few examples so we can see how these exchanges occur and what the results were. Many call it faith healing, but it generally seems to be transmisison of low level bio-photons requiring very close contact with a patient.

Faith-Healing

In actual fact, in so far as faith-healing is concerned, religion is not all that important. There are numerous cases of faith-healers performing their faith-healing acts without using religion at all. A case in point is the science of hypnotism, the practice of which involves no religious aspects at all. Those who associate religion with faith-healing are in a way engaging in a subtle form of illusion trying to attract converts to their particular religion by making use of faith healing and describing certain cures as miraculous acts.

The methods employed by faith healers are to condition the minds of patients into having a certain mental attitude with the result that certain favorable psychological and physiological changes invariably take place. This attracts the condition of the mind, the heart, the consequent blood circulation and other related organic functions of the body, thus creating a feeling of a sense of well-being. If sickness is attributed to the condition of the mind, then the mind can certainly be properly conditioned to assist in eradicating whatever illness that may occur.

In this context, it is to be noted that the constant and regular practice of meditation can help to minimize, if not to completely eradicate, various forms of illnesses. There are many discourses in the Teaching of the Buddha where it was indicated that various forms of sicknesses were eradicated through the conditioning of the mind. Thus, it is worthwhile to practice meditation in order to attain mental and physical well-being.

Ruptured Disk Cure-The patient had a ruptured disk that caused him unending pain. A coworker performed hands on healing which caused a feeling of great heat. The pain left and returned 5 times before finally having ALL PAIN completely removed. After returning to the doctor it was determined that the ruptured disk had miraculously healed!

Lost Leg Pain-This same coworker helped another who had lost a leg in the Vietnam War. The healer prayed and laid his hands on the patient and in 5 minutes the hurting area was very hot. After one treatment, pain that had been had for 20 years was gone.

Skin Cancer-A melanoma was eliminated within one day by this same faith healer and was a visible testimony of the success of this work.

Cat Healing-No Placebo effect for sure here as a stupid cat was cured in one hands-on-session that was almost certainly going to die.

Traiteur Healing-It is common in Louisiana Cajun culture to have persons who have the gift of healing, thought to be a blessing from God, but those who practiced this ancient "ART" seemed to have been too young to understand what they were doing when they started healing. These special people are known as *traiteurs*, [Similar to the 'powow' healer of the Pennsylvania German community or the 'power doctor' in the Ozarks] They do not advertise their powers and never take money.

Buddha Healing-In Tibetan Buddhism faith healers are said to be given the "gift" from Buddha. About the same as the Christian healing, there seems to be a difference about what "faith" is. While that is not a subject of this book, let's look at the New Testament to see how it worked back then.

New Testament

God has given us 42 clear examples in Bible texts of the exercise of this E-M message healing with one's hands. Careful study reveals a very clear pattern that definitely shows and exalts the supernatural nature of true Christian healing. Let us now look at the people who were healed. They were people from every walk of life. One of the most startling facts is that many of them did not particularly have faith in the healer. In John 9 Jesus healed a blind man whom He met in passing. <u>The blind man did not even know who He was.</u> A similar instance is shown in Luke 13:12. In Acts 3:2-8 the beggar <u>did not have any idea what Peter was going to do</u>. In Acts 28:8 Publius' father lay sick of a fever so he could not have been healed by hypnotic suggestion. Many times, <u>a man was delirious from fever </u>or extended sickness. This all points us to E-M messaging directed from the healer's body.

Bad Faith Healers-By this we might understand something about <u>faith healers that say the reason some are not cured is that THE PATIENT did not believe</u>. If you noticed from my examples, many of those healed by the "original" faith healers <u>had no "faith" at all in the healing</u>.

I think this is an important thing. Faith Healing does not require Faith- in God it only need hands that do something.

When hands are placed on bodies, there seems to be some type of energy that is transferred. If this emission is focused, it can help neutralize incorrect photonic emissions in the body of the person receiving bio-photons from the healer. There is a possibility we can learn more from other verses as we have read about some individuals emitting so much E-M/ Photon energy that they glow.

Bio-Photonic Halo

If you remember from Religious histories, there was mention of Bioluminescence or HALOs. Certainly, there is evidence that a concentration of bio-photonic energy could be sent through a body to help cure people, but if someone really became "charged with faith" the Bible indicated that the person would glow. The glow was most noticeable around the face as many wore clothes so it looked like their head had a Halo. We are told Noah was born with this type of radiance, and Adam reportedly had this glow. Angels covered their faces to keep people from recognizing the glow and then there was Moses. When Moses came down off the mountaintop after talking with God, he was "glowing" and had one of these halos as bio-photons were emitted in huge amounts.

*Exodus 34:29-35-Now it was so, when Moses came down from Mount Sinai--that Moses did not know that **the skin of his face shone** while he talked with Him. So, when Aaron and all the children of Israel saw Moses, behold, the **skin of his face shone**, and they were afraid to come near him. And when Moses had finished speaking with them, he put a veil on his face. But whenever Moses went in before the LORD to speak with Him, he would take the veil off until he came* *out; and he would come out and speak to the children of Israel whatever he had been commanded. And whenever the children of Israel saw the face of Moses, that the **skin of Moses' face shone**, then Moses <u>would put the veil on his face</u> again, until he went in to speak with Him.*

He must have been scary and I'm certain he could have introduced a substantial amount of the correct bio-photons into someone to cure them. The image below left may give us an idea what Moses might have looked like. The image right shows and artist's rendition. I know you are thinking he could write at night with his built-in night light, but, that is just a joke.

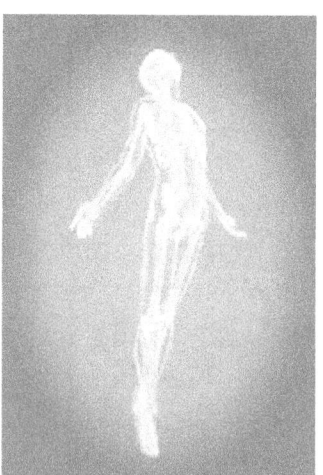 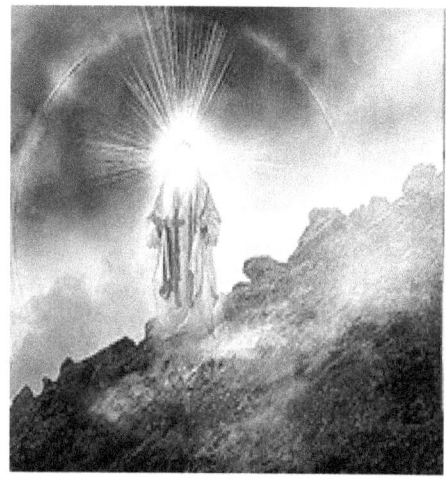

Today, scientists are finding out this is a truth that needs to be considered as very low levels of invisible and visible light are both emitted from the body and during times of stress or disease, this output is increased. Besides the emissions, all organic life absorbs and processes light. Bio-photon emission or spontaneous ultra-weak light emission has been observed from almost all living organisms, with intensities ranging from 10^{-19} to 10^{-16} W/cm^2. A number of studies also found that emissions change by various cycles of the body. In Moses case, His head turned bluish. Possibly his whole body was the same, but most was already covered. In the case of Moses, his body had a halo. This happened without Moses direction as the Heart has a separate consciousness.

Heart Consciousness

As I mentioned, the heart brain, may well be more conscious of the "environment than our head-Brain. Certainly, the heart is more aware of the soul and spirit as it interfaces with both according to the Biblical testimony.

This is because, the Heart not only filters information from our consciousness, but also from our free-floating Soul and the intra-universe communicating spirit [This part of our existence sort of to Heaven and back]. Additionally, it seems the intimate association of feelings appears to be supported much more by the Heart brains than our head brain. There is a verse in Proverbs written by a man that was supposedly the wisest man, ever. Solomon's words tell us what we will learn in this book.

Proverbs 4:23 *Above all else, guard your heart, for everything you do flows from it.*

Introspective Awareness

There is now an idea of "introspective awareness" of the heart itself. Possibly you can say we are conversing when only you, your head brain and your heart brain are in the room. While this is the scientific rage, I am more inclined to think that the soul uses the heart-brain to communicate with others. As we remove our self-centered emotion to the emotion of love and protection of others, our soul becomes very powerful [increase primary faith] according to Biblical teachings. This will make more sense as we go along.

Heart-Brain Photonic Messaging Sight

Some scientists have described the Heart-brain as having some type of vision and Biblical verses confirm this attitude. What scientists have found is that that sees at a much lower wavelength than our Eyes, but it does sense electro-magnetic [E-M] waves just like our eyes. This is an exciting component of our Heart brain and it associated efforts. What the Heart sees is stress, love, hope, understanding and tension from the Heart brains of other individuals nearby. These things help the heart generate messages to help heal those around us. Our heart sends out messages to calm of stress the environment and it receives this same indication from others nearby. It has been long known that if you place individuals together if more are hostile, soon almost all with take on that feeling and vice versa. A calm or pleasant emission will make other conform to that calmness or goodness. This is a great responsibility. Smile at those you pass by as smiling helps trigger he good E-M transmissions.

The Heart's Electro-Magnetic Field-Research has also revealed that the heart communicates information to the brain and throughout the body via electromagnetic field interactions. Sort-of like the DNA sends messages to adjacent cells, the Heart sends messages to the brain other parts of the body, and nearby entities.

The heart generates the body's most powerful and most extensive rhythmic electromagnetic field. The heart's magnetic messaging <u>can be detected several feet away from the body.</u>

It was proposed that; this heart field acts as a carrier wave for information that provides a global synchronizing signal for the entire body.

Ephesians 1:18 *-the <u>**eyes of your heart**</u> may be enlightened*

When we look at Proverbs 15:30 we see that if someone comes near another's Heart-brain, the brain can sense/see if the person is filled with the spirit/light or not.

Proverbs 15:30 *Light in a messenger's eyes brings <u>joy to the heart.</u>*

While the heart emissions are most noticeable outside the body, our head-brain is continuously messaging and working its miracles with all type of E-M/photonic messages. Fortunately or unfortunately, because the brain is this massive E-M communication hub, it can be manipulated.

What Do Bio-Photons Do?

I think I might have lost some of you who have believed that light was made up of these tiny particles vibrating at different rates to make colors we see and all this E-M waves, and life affecting life, and all the rest is just mystic who-ha. Let me back up again and try to tie things together and see how photonic messaging is beginning to allow us to understand our bodies.

As Moses stated in Genesis, Bio-Photons produces or establishes life. OK! He actually inferred that light was life, but hopefully you are opening your mind to why he would suggest such a thing. It explains how enzymes can recognize their respective substrates, how antibodies in the immune system can grab onto specific foreign invaders and disarm them. By extension, that's how proteins can 'dock' with different partner proteins, or latch onto specific nucleic acids to control gene expression, or assemble into ribosomes for translating proteins, or other multi-molecular complexes that modify the genetic messages in various ways.

While I have not been getting into too much detail in this book, let me again say, at the basic level of how light miraculously appears; E-M waves enter our eyes, cause the rods and cones to active, and E-M signals are transferred, mostly by nerves, to the head brain where message decoding establishes what we call visibility, but the eyes are only a tiny part of the body that uses, transmits, and decodes E-M emissions.

It seems that <u>somehow</u> each molecule <u>sends out a unique electro-magnetic emission</u> that can "sense" the field of the complimentary molecule. By this, molecules recognize their particular targets and vice versa by electro-magnetic resonance. In other words, the molecules send out specific frequencies of electro-magnetic waves which, not only enable them <u>to 'see'</u> each other, but also <u>to influence</u> each other at a distance and become drawn to each other. With about 100,000 chemical reactions happening in every cell each second and each one initiated by some special coding of bio-photonic emissions, you can see that photonic energy is switching on and off continuously. One researcher put it this way---

"We are swimming in an ocean of light."--- Just like Moses tried to say 3500 years ago.

It has been suggested that the way DNA is coiled is to allow it to change its "resonance" to send and receive various frequencies needed to support life.

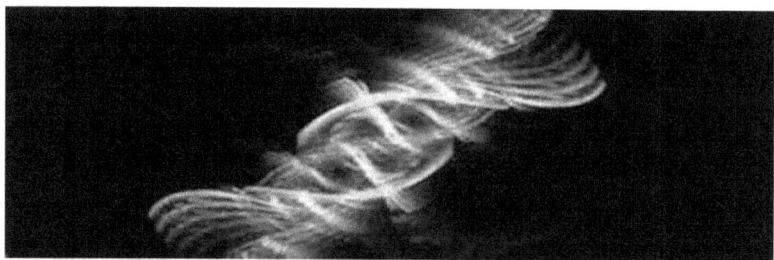

As shown above, like a tiny spring, higher frequencies would have DNA tighten while low frequency emission needs would have DNA loosen its coils to "resonate" and allow better transmission at the lower frequencies.

Here is a strange thing. It is also known that as the DNA uncoils, the amount of light emitted is increased.

We now can sense what happens when you get a cut or scratch on your skin. The images following show the extra photonic activity in areas of distress on our skin and anywhere else on or in our bodies. This is not just light. It is a message carried in the light. It is a real change in the characteristics of the skin cells.

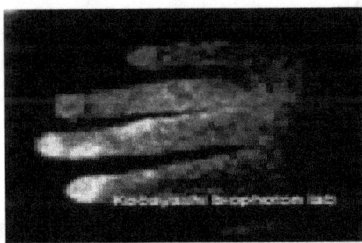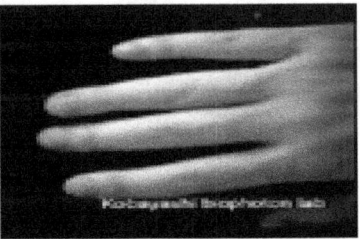

When speaking of real change, commercials tell us how cancer is going away with drugs, chemotherapy, blasting X-Rays, and all sorts of things. One would think from these commercials that soon all cancer will be eradicated and no one would need to go to the Hospital.

If cancer is to be controlled, it is going to be by E-M Waves.

So, our DNA, tells a cut to reconstruct itself and DNA tells us when came in contact with stinging nettle and poison is introduced. DNA tells us to wrinkle our skin or make a mole and on-and on. When it comes to cancer, DNA has its part as well.

Deadly Cancer

If someone has told you we are beginning to understand and destroy cancer so people will live longer, they are not telling you the truth.

Cancer is Increasing in America

As shown below of cancer death rates of men and women in almost all areas. The first column is total cancer deaths of men and the second one if the total for women. Followed by that are deaths from breast cancer, Prostate cancer, and colon cancer of men and women. Certainly, if we, as a society began placing our hands on the sick and actually believe that the messages produced would heal patients, there could be a curing, but it really requires us to use our Heart-brain messaging more effectively. Instead, our cutting, radiation chemo-therapy and all the rest are not working.

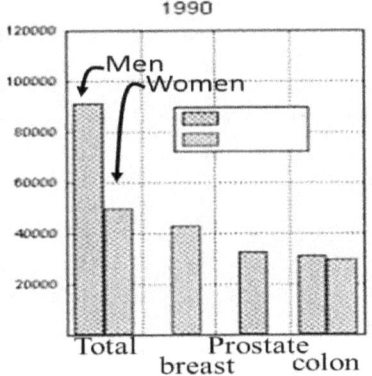

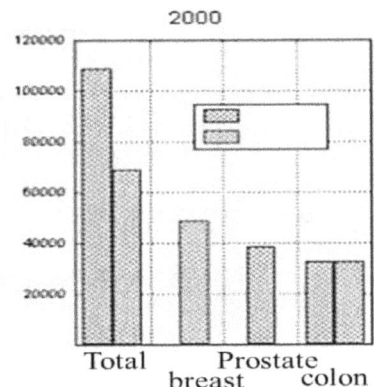

Almost all major cancers have INCREASED with about 180 thousand deaths in 2000 as opposed to about 130 thousand for these 4 cancer types alone in 1990.

That's almost a 40% Increase in Death in a 10-year ADVANCEMENT cycle.

Seems we are trying to increase death rather than trying to control death forming issues. Around the world we find the same thing with the United States having about ¼ of the deaths from cancers as the total rest of the world's high-income countries.

High-income countries

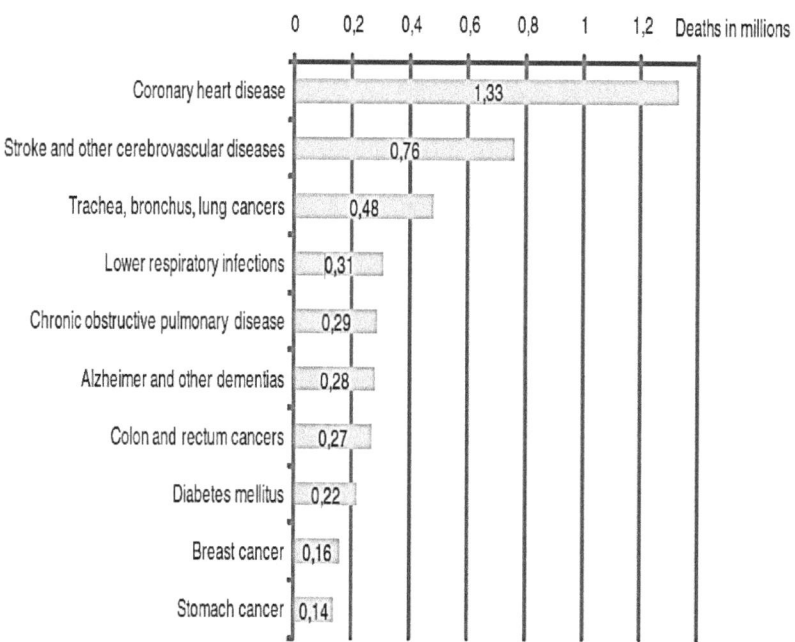

	Deaths in millions
Coronary heart disease	1,33
Stroke and other cerebrovascular diseases	0,76
Trachea, bronchus, lung cancers	0,48
Lower respiratory infections	0,31
Chronic obstructive pulmonary disease	0,29
Alzheimer and other dementias	0,28
Colon and rectum cancers	0,27
Diabetes mellitus	0,22
Breast cancer	0,16
Stomach cancer	0,14

Drugs haven't worked, early detection hasn't worked, self-examination hasn't worked, and colonoscopies <u>haven't worked.</u> The biggest one you should know is radiation, chemotherapy, and focused radiations <u>haven't worked</u>. They are only used to allow for larger hospitals to be built. I'm not one who is against trying everything we can to halt disease; especially cancer that took my precious daughter in 2014, but we had better get an understanding of cancer and other cellular modifying diseases quickly or we will have to build many more hospitals to prolong the lives of those infected.

Surgery Isn't the Answer

The only thing that seems to help for a time is cutting huge chucks out of our bodies. If we start understanding what cells are and how they work we will be able to do something and that is where bio-photonics comes in. This book deals with all types of investigations, experiments, treatments and homeopathy dealing not only with bio-photonic use to remove the threat of cancer, but in almost every single issue we have today with our bodies. Most of these things deal with the elimination of yanking out big pieces of our body as a form of treatment. Doctors and scientists are now <u>trying to talk to cancer</u> with bio-photonic messages and it's starting to work.

One absolutely understandable science being used today deals with <u>bio-photonics</u> in a somewhat different way. They call it Ultraviolet-Blood-Irradiation.

Ultraviolet Blood Irradiation

UV Blood irradiation or UBI [photonic messaging] has been around since before the 1900s but it is done in a cleaner environment today. This seems somewhat similar to a process called Chelation that would pull out your blood and remove heavy metals before redepositing the lighter blood. This process is totally associated with LIGHT changing cells. In this case Blood is yanked out of your body and irradiated with UV light. UV light kills germs; how it does it will be discussed at a later time, but the UV light irradiated blood is then slowly returned to the body while other blood is removed and irradiated and put back until all the blood has been cycled through the UV bacteria killer. The next image shows a typical session where a patient is connected to the irradiator by way of a tube bringing blood.

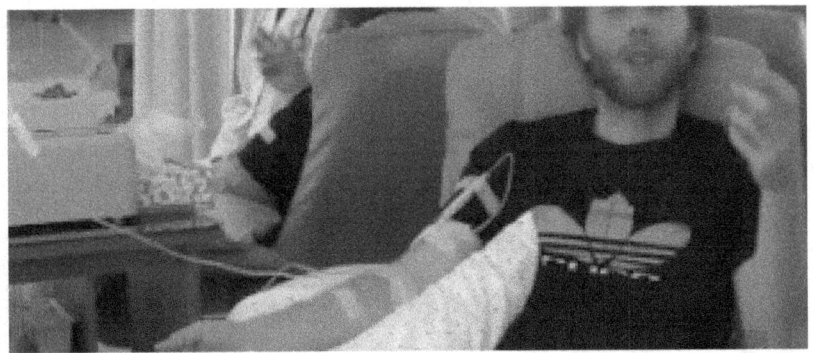

Low and behold, all types of illness began to be helped. While most was done by the elimination of bad germs and bateria, it seems that the irradiated blood transmits photonic massages in the UV to adjacent cells which aid in the healing process. We know this not only because the success of UBI treatments, but also from other work to be discussed. When I say it is helping patients with diseases, here is a short list of those affected in a positive way:

- Kills bacteria and viruses in the blood and super charges the immune system

- Improves circulation and oxygenation to tissues

- Balances Hormones and other necessary chemicals and transmitters in the body

- Increases the body's tolerance towards radiation or chemotherapy

- Heightens anti-inflammatory factors in the body

- Works as a powerful anti-infective agent

- Reduces tissue pain

- Cardiovascular protection through increased metabolism of cholesterol, uric acid, and glucose

This bio-photonic process aids in treatment of Asthma, Allergies, Chronic Fatigue, Chronic Yeast Infection, Fibromyalgia, Heart Disease, Hepatitis, Lupus, Non-healing Wounds, Poor Circulation, Respiratory Infection, Rheumatoid Arthritis, Shingles, Staph Infections, Lyme Disease, Flu, Viral Infections, Fungal Infections, bronchitis, sinusitis, tuberculosis, pneumonia, Cancer, septicemia, peritonitis, polio, encephalitis, mumps, measles, mononucleosis, herpes, Hepatitis C, HIV, thrombophlebitis, diabetic ulcers, overwhelming toxemias, delayed union of fractures, MS, and others.

All this is done with light.

While this is not the answer for cancer, it seems to be a good start. Maybe investigating this stuff will be useful so let's go a little deeper and see where this came from.

Ultraviolet Germicidal Irradiation

Discovered in 1878 by a man named A. Downes ultraviolet light seems to kill bacteria. If the UV has a sufficiently short wavelength, 250 to 254 nm, called UV-C, microorganisms including bacteria, virus, and larger parasites all lost the capability to reproduce and their DNA began to disintegrate. A typical UV-C emitter is shown below.

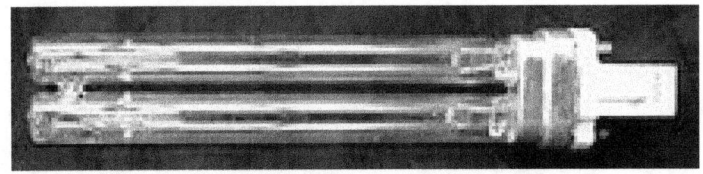

Initially, it looked like the UV blasted the cells and destroyed them, but a newer view suggests that the UV-C message to the cells is one that tells the cell to kill itself.

When the message is received, nucleic acids in these organisms that make DNA are disrupted, leaving them unable to perform vital cellular functions. The bug is history.

As demonstrated in the first section, the trick might be getting the UV-C into the blood. As a strange phenomenon, tiny bacteria and viruses as harder to "disable" than larger parasites like cryptosporidium. It was determined that as animals become more complex, their sensitivity to bio-photonic interactions was more direct and actually required a lower dose for inactivation of the animal or parasite.

We were beginning to understand that photons and E-M waves could control, damage, and even kill cells, but some would question how the photons could be transferred. Did cells emit photons?????

Kurlian Photography

If you hadn't read the introduction and I told you people send out photons from their cells would that seem odd? Kurlian photography is not a "true" indicator of bio-photonic emission, but it is well known and may have been responsible for early studies so let's just take a quick look. These odd images were photographed showing what had been defined as an aura as shown below from hands, leaves freshly picked and metal objects. Let me tell you the metal is not alive so there is something else going on. The images below are some that are typically shown.

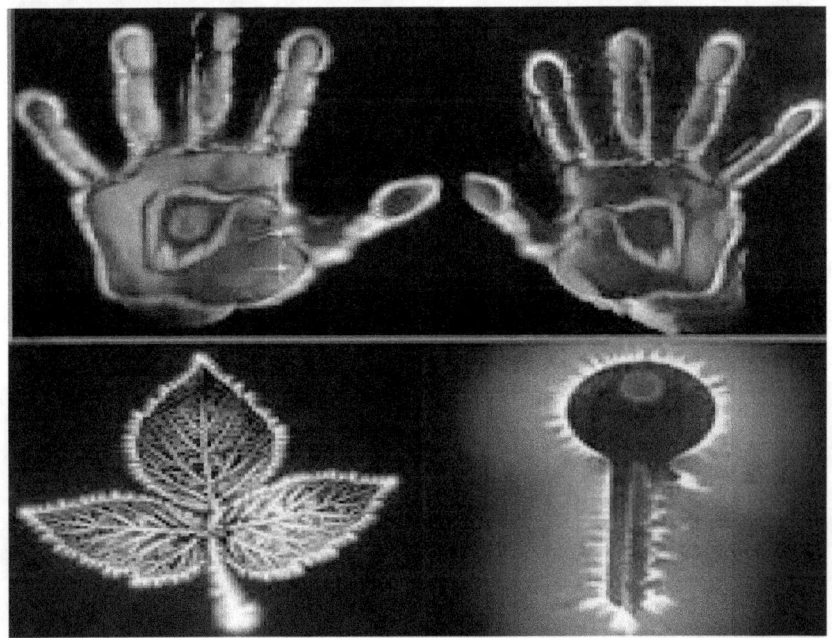

Generally speaking, if there is a difference in potential and a very high voltage, there will be a generation of electromagnetic fields. Notice that the metal provided a larger "HALO" than the living objects, As we can expect, EM fields can be built with highly conductive metals better than with live objects, however, the emissions from people and leaves were disturbing in that there was a clear sign of emission of some sort as a cut leaf would try to emit to the missing part and the halo extends past portions that had been ripped away as shown below.

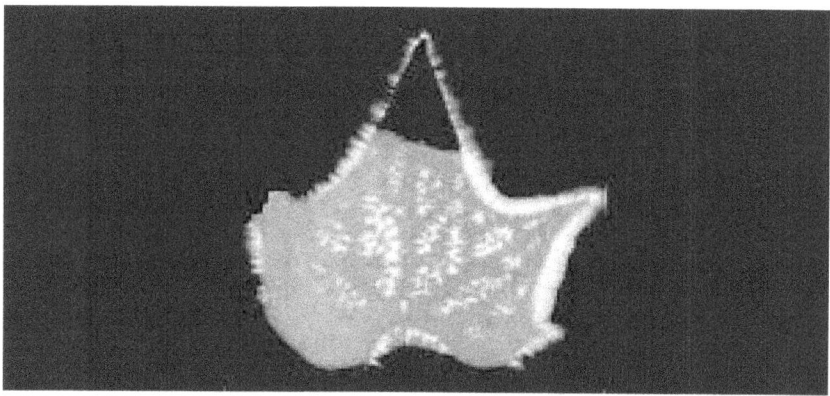

Later, we will find that photonic emissions of plants and animals are the exact opposites. What we will be finding is that these opposite emissions might be the very thing to fix us. We will get to that later, but right now let's see what happens when people lose sunlight.

Bio-photon Communication

The bio-photons are used for internal chemical reactions and also for communication with the internal and external environments. So, when an electron in the atom drops from a higher to lower energy level it emits a photon or what may also be considered an "information pack". It is believed that each atom responds to a specific light frequency. The atom absorbs some of the light during what is called an electron quantum change and reflects some the light for communication with its environment. The same process has been seen at a larger level in the molecules.

Each cell in our body contains over 100,000 chemical reactions per second. We give birth to approximately 10,000,000 cells per second and an equivalent amount die in that period of time, so there is a lot of opportunity to make photons.

It's not that straight forward. It is believed that our consciousness affects the production the bio-photons within the atom. Somehow, photons are amplified and reduced by mood, stress, Chi and/or something called faith. The light produced by each atom plays a critical part in supporting the chemical reactions in the network of new cells. Overall, the study of bio-photon communication within the body is still in its early stages. In our infancy, we are now beginning to understand the importance of coherent light oscillation within the body for its proper function. The image below shows emissions in the morning and later in the day.

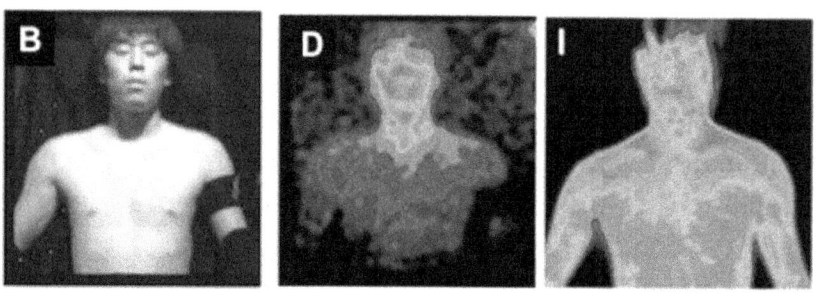

People emit more photonic energy in the middle of the day.

The following image shows the emissions of a leaf in the morning [D] and later in the day [E and F]. While the peak seems different, there is no question of emission and cycle of both animal and plant life.

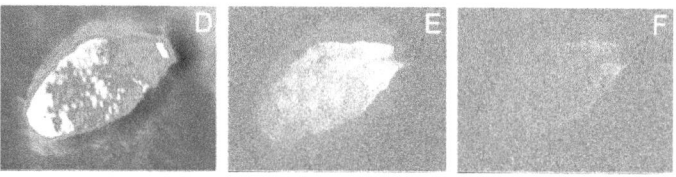

Plants do better in the morning.

One reason we emit more light throughout the day is we absorb more. Studies have tried to see if this absorption can give us indications of bio-photonic treatments.

Winter Phenomenon

Everyone knows there is less light in the winter and more light in the summer. The question is, with less light, would there be more medical issues and Bio-phonons are not recharged as they would during summer months??? If we look at the chart below we can see that the answer is yes. Every winter, all sorts of disorders increase until the sun comes out again.

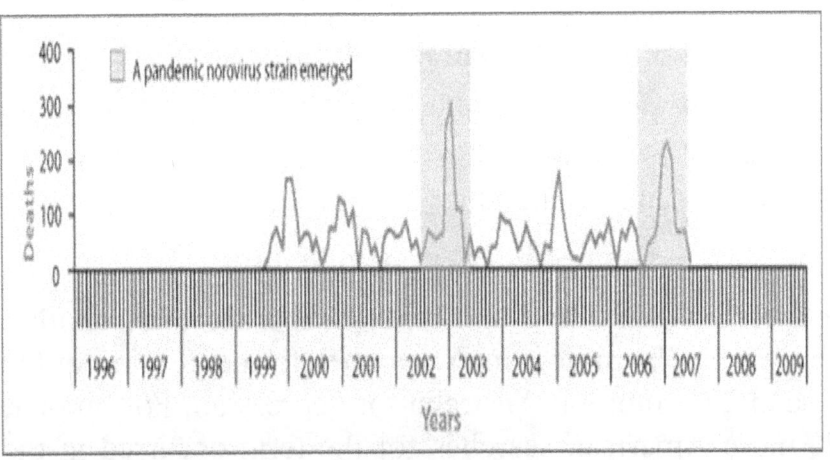

We get sicker in the Winter because we don't absorb as much light.

American Journal of Preventive Medicine indicated the following: "*All mental health queries followed seasonal patterns with winter peaks and summer troughs.*" They found that mental health queries in general were 14% higher in the winter in the U.S. and 11% higher in the Australian winter.

Schizophrenia Worse in Winter

The seasonal timing of queries regarding each disorder was also similar in the two countries. In both countries, eating disorders and schizophrenia surged during winter months; those in the U.S. were 37% more likely and Australians were 42% more likely to seek information about these disorders during colder weather than during the summer. And compared to summer searches, schizophrenia queries were 37% more common in the American winter and 36% more frequent during the Australian winter.

ADHD Worse in Winter

ADHD queries were also highly seasonal, with 31% more winter searches in the U.S. and 28% more in Australia compared to summer months.

Depression Worse in Winter

Searches for depression and bipolar disorder were similar. There were 19% more winter searches for depression in the U.S. and 22% more in Australia for depression. For bipolar, 16% more American searches for the term occurred in the winter than in the summer, and 18% more searches occurred during the Australian winter.

Previous research suggests that shorter daylight hours and the social isolation that accompanies harsh weather conditions might explain <u>some of these seasonal differences in mental illnesses</u> but not all Vitamin D was also thought about, but similarly, not recharging our photon emitters just like plants seems to be the more reasonable cause of increased mental illness.

Suicide Worse in Winter

Searches for 'suicide' were 29% more common in winter in America and 24% more common during the colder season in Australia, other investigations showed that completed suicides tend to peak in spring and early summer after the reduction in sunlight had done its work.

Wintertime SAD

As it effects over 5% of our population, you've probably heard about seasonal affective disorder, or SAD. SAD typically causes depression [sorry for the play on words] as the days get shorter and colder.

Many disorders are much worse in the Winter.

Let's Add Photons

All bodies are made of cells, tissue, and organs which communicate how to function as a body. There is a hope that light treatments will assist in intercellular and intracellular communication. It is suggested that with some type of photon centric treatment method, ALL bodies will improve their ability to heal themselves. Depending on what stage of degeneration the body is in will determine the impact and effect the treatments will have, as well as what the individual does to promote their long- term outcomes of better mind, body, soul, and spirit health. Here is what researcher Dr. Fritz Popp had to say about this important topic.

> *"We now know, for example, that light can initiate, or arrest, reactions in the cells, and that genetic cellular damage can be virtually repaired, within hours, by faint beams of light. We are still on the threshold of fully understanding the complex relationship between light and life, but we can now say, emphatically that <u>the function of our entire metabolism is dependent on light.</u> This radiation from living cells, or bio-photon emission, represents a regulating energy field that encompasses the entire organism and affects the entire body's biochemical processes."*

That being said the first attempt is something called color-puncture.

Color-Puncture

Instead of sticking pins in your skin, why not just push photons into th eskin cells.

One attempt at using color light to save us is something called color-puncture. Similar to Accupuncture, this deals with photons. It is a holistic healing and one of Europe's most popular healing disciplines. The originator of Color-puncture is a German scientist, acupuncturist and naturopath named Peter Mandel who conducted over 25 years of intensive "empirical research" to develop this unique system of healing. Color-puncture involves focusing colored light on acupuncture points on the skin in order to energize powerful healing impulses in our physical and energy bodies. The images below show special feet, hands, and face color-puncture type devices.

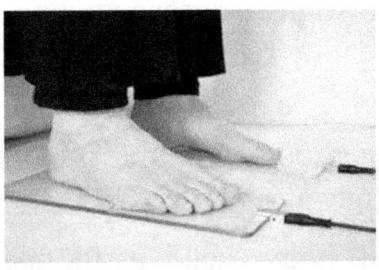 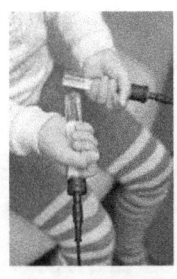 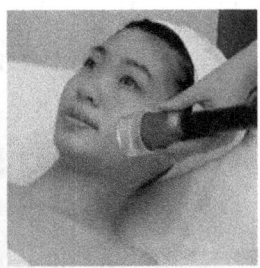

If you are really into it, more sestablished color theapists have massive colormachines to emit into your cells the life giving photons.

Skin Rejuvenation

Bio-photonic Light Therapy is on the rise and it seems to offer a vast quantity of benefits for skin. There are a number of different color wavelengths that help the skin in a positive yet different ways. The layers of the skin are comprised of a high content of blood and water which allows them to easily and readily absorb and accept light. Once absorbed into the skin the different colors work jhard offering their ownunique benefits. Bio-photonic Light Therapy is safe and healthy and has no negative side effects.

- **Blue light** seems to reduce p-acne bacteria. It can get through many skin layers, so there is little reddening of the skin.

- **Green light**, however, can go slightly deeper and helps in melanine production and redusces unwanted pigmentations

- **Red lights** increases callagen production, and provides essential energy for celular renewal

The following images are for full body "help" as the main photonic emission of the body is red, most of these treatments seems to be with red light, but facial treatments are certainly looking into the blue and green levels.

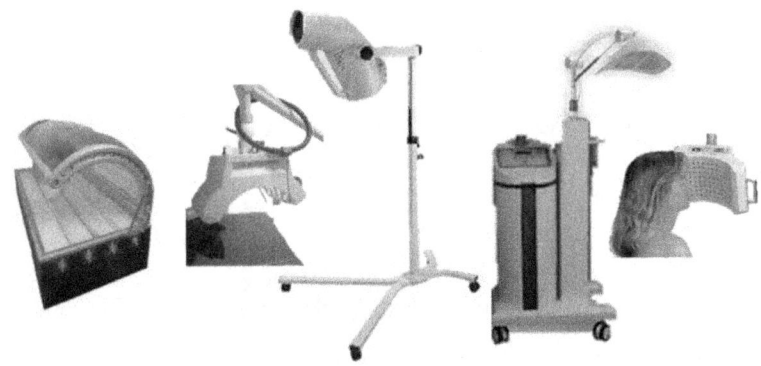

Patients report not only changes in their bodies, but improved emotional outlooks and a clearer sense of life direction after treatments. Patients usually report the following:

- Skin looking younger
- Fine lines gone
- Tightening of skin
- Less blemishes, Rosacea, and redness
- Faster burn scar reduction
- Less Eczema, Psoriasis

This gives us a good Segway into the next color treatment. For this we start with rocks.

Chakra Balancing

I must confess that I have studied various levels of attuneness of our mind and soul with something called universal resonance, but as far as I can determine, Bio-Photonics has little to do with the characterization of Chakra levels of awareness. That has not kept "practitioners from laying different color rocks at locations associated with levels of consciousness as shown below.

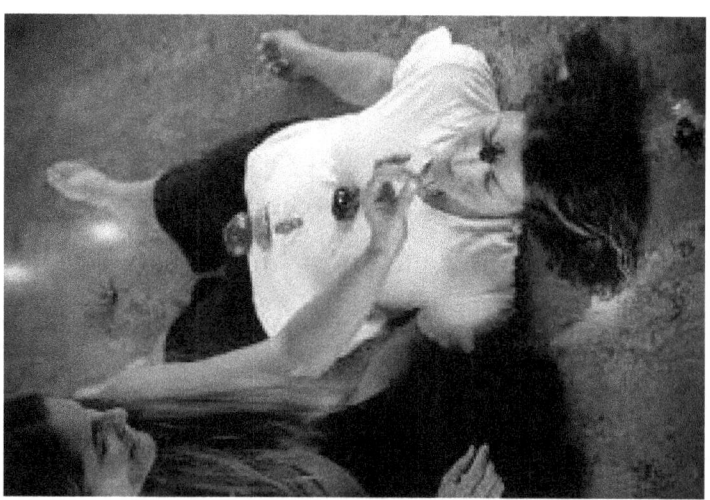

It seems that the rocks just laid there and the patient was still sick.

Whith the new craze of bio-Photonics, the colored stones are now changed to colored lights.

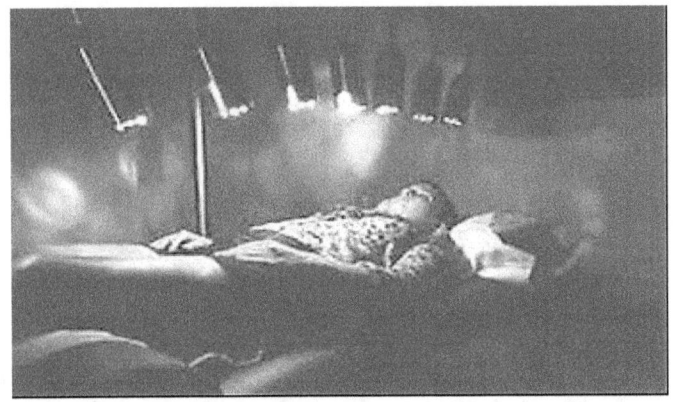

- **Red** for sexual need and focus,
- **Orange** for self awarenes and egocentricity,
- **Yellow** for Survival and the understanding of the world,
- **Green** for the Heart and love of others.
- **Light blue** for selfless love and self actualization,
- **Dark Blue** for the third eye awareness of our universe and reality, and
- **Violet** for the crown chakra for awareness between universes.

The light wavelengths seem to to be more due to the color stones that were used previously. This is supposed to allow you to meditate more fully, but I'm having trouble with the science. In Anthropic science, these levels of awareness are dependednt on a common consciousness and the ability to interact with light. This light is not the same thing as photons but that is a totally different subject. Let be get back to bio-photonics, what it is, how it works, what it can do for us and how it affects the entire world. That is enough for a single book.

Depression and Light

I know I am sort of making fun of the turn light bulbs on treatment method, but there is at least one study that shows massive introduction of light does reduce depression, so we had better, at least, look. The first chart below describes a 10-patient study using a standard called the Hamilton Depression Rating [HAM-D]. The second is similar in that the same 10 people were also evaluated by the Hamilton Anxiety Rating Scale [HAM-A],

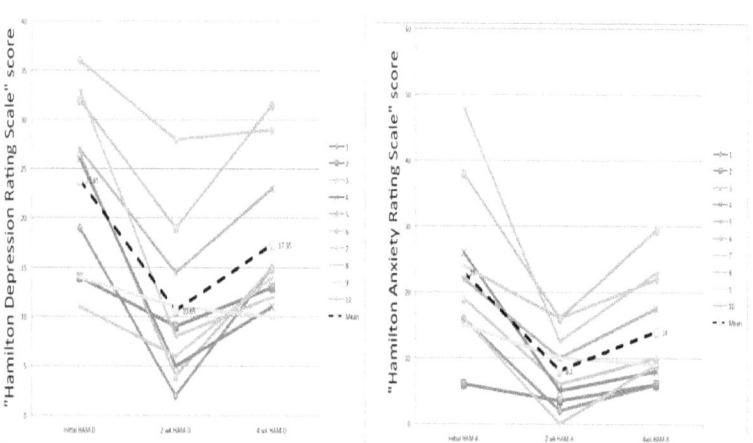

The test included a series of photon bombardments on the skull, but the details are not known to me. What is evident is that the particular lights used worked. The huge dips in the middle show massive reductions in depression and

anxiety. The slight increases at the end show that even after 4 weeks, the symptoms were still under much better control.

The Mean percentage reductions [the dashed lines in the charts] in HAM-D scores were 54.3% better at 2 weeks post-treatment and 27.1% at 4-weeks post-treatment. All 10 patients were "improvers," defined in the literature as those patients who respond to an intervention for depression with at least a 20% reduction in HAM-D. The HAM-A results were similar and even more impressive.

HAM sounds like hands, so let's see how hands might be affected by bio-photonics.

Bio-Photonics So Far

Hopefully, you have started to understand the details presented as bio-photons can save your life, help you help others, allow for better understanding of people and plants, and possibly give us different direction for communication with others. So far, we have seen the following:

- Light is associated with all life. This includes bacteria, plants, and animals.

- Without light there is no life. Even after death there seems to be this outward indication of life for some time as bio-photons continue to emit.

- Even after the death of plants, these emissions can aid in fighting disease if they are not cooked. This can be done by injection, ingesting, or possibly even by rubbing.

- We can make a general statement that Cancer is too few coherent biophotons and a huge bio-photonic output that is in some disorder. Cancer should be able to be treated by modifying the emissions.

- If plants were organically grown before being harvested, they seem to output more healing light. The following image shows the difference in organic mushrooms and commercially grown ones. To me it looks like organic food could help us more.

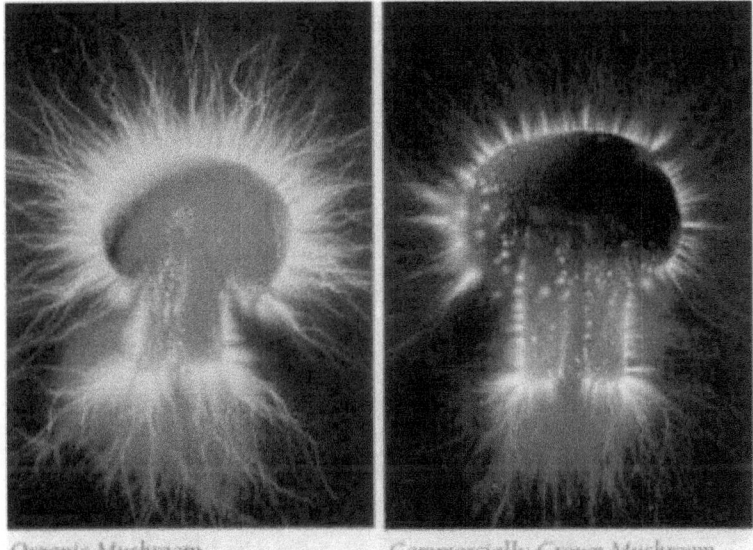

Organic Mushroom   Commercially Grown Mushroom

- If one <u>does not have major issues</u> in his body like cancer, light emissions in the tested areas will be low. Cancer seems to increase bio-photonic emission in the stressed area so we can locate cancer easier.
- Everybody has a halo of very low intensity light.

Type of Emissions

Highest visible energy levels emitted by humans are 470-570 nm. This means that if one had enough people in a dark enough area and they were stressed, there would be a tiny blue haze that could be recognized. That being said, there are many wavelengths emitted by the cells as shown in the next graphic. The ones being studied the most are UV, Infrared, and Visible emissions, but notice there are many others to test that could affect how we optically communicate between our own cells and with our environment. Looks like we emit quite a few radio stations and even some X-rays. One can imagine that Moses could not go near a radio or TV set without messing them up.

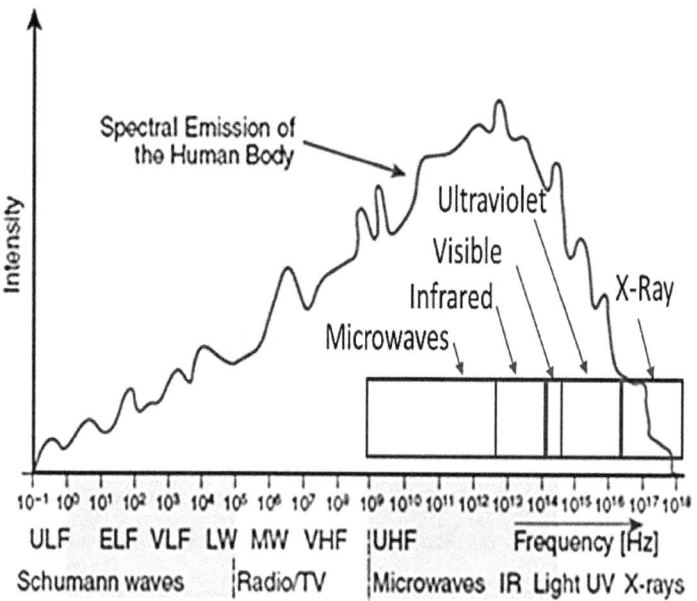

With all this emitting, do we need to turn ourselves off occasionally? The answer seems to make me yawn.

Sleep and Sex

Have you ever wondered why we seem to need sleep? Some have indicated people need to have the brain think and coordinate inputs from the day. I know it sounded stupid, but they told you anyway. Why wouldn't the brain do that better when you were awake? While there are no studies on this topic, let me tell you what I think is a more reasonable requirement for turning off the lights and shutting down the entrance of light to the brain.

Pineal

Called the third eye, the pineal gland seems to have similar structure to the eye [similar E-M field receptors] except it is located in the center of the skull and is <u>bathed with more blood that any other organ.</u> One thing we know is that the Pineal gland wakes when we are asleep and manufactures something called melatonin which aids in our sleep. Some researchers now believe that the pineal <u>may direct cell bio-photonic emissions</u> in some way and this melatonin may also help regulate Electro-Magnetic emissions and interpretation of bio-photonic communications. We can believe from the massive amount of blood circulating through this gland that it is extremely important to the body and we have little knowledge of what it does today, but we have some data.

Pineal Glands in many non-mammalian vertebrates have a strong resemblance to the photoreceptor cells of the eye.

Some evolutionary biologists believe that the pineal cells share a common were the ancestor to retina E-M sensor cells in the eye.

In some animals, exposure to light of this gland can change the animal's biorhythm.

Some early vertebrate fossil skulls <u>have a pineal opening</u> so that it probably had some vision characteristic.

The lamprey and the tuatara both have this same type of pineal opening and this thing is photosensitive. The structures appear to include cornea, lens and retina.

The pineal gland is weird in that it has profuse blood flow, second only to the kidney, so we can be sure that it once was of great importance. While doctors are perplexed at why this insignificant gland would need so much blood, it is obvious that whatever happened 6 thousand years ago made the extra blood flow unnecessary.

The brain of a Cretaceous Period bird was found with a large parietal eye and pineal gland so it's been used for some time now to provide additional insight beyond normal visual E-M sensing of the Eyes.

Production of melatonin by the pineal gland is stimulated by darkness and inhibited by light. This melatonin stuff affects sex drive as we will examine.

OK! We have a tiny organ that used to be huge and it used to be an aid in seeing, regulating moods and sex drive, but our bodies are still trying to supply it with enough blood to run a huge organ. Today the tiny little thing seems to have been abandoned by our bodies, but maybe we just can't "see" what it can do.

Pineal and Sex

Besides melatonin it regulates our sex hormones which aid in our understanding of "self" [Self desire, desire for the opposite sex, lust, love, and all the rest]. While I'm on this subject let me quickly discuss something with you that has little to do with photons but a lot to do with health of the body. That is one of the most reactive substances on the planet known as Fluorine.

Fluorine from fluorinated water is now being found in large amounts in the pineal gland. This reactive substance seems to trigger sex hormone levels and introduce puberty earlier such that children have not been able to develop an understanding of sexual difference. Some suggest that this is increasing the homosexual deviation in our society. Here are a few studies. [The * indicates high fluorination before the study]

- **Canada** –in a 1988 study-**2%** of the tested population were determined to be homosexual or bisexual.

- **UK**- In a 2010 study with little fluorination- **1.5%** were gay or bisexual.

- **Australia***-In a 2014 study- about **3.5%** of men and women were identified as being homosexual or bisexual.

- **Ireland***- In a 2006 study- **6%** were determined to be bisexual or homosexual.

- **New Zealand***- In a 2007 study- **4%** were homosexual or bisexual.

- **USA***- In a 2011 study- **4%** were gay or bisexual.

Fluorinated water seems to increase or even double the amount of sexual confusion in a society by causing the collection of fluorine in the Pineal Glands before puberty.

If we run the numbers of individuals now having "Erectile Dysfunction" early in life, it also seems to correlate with the increases in the fluorine in the Pineal. We could possibly find similar statistics on prepubescent sex, but the data would be hard to gather. Sorry for the diversion, but, we really have not studied the Pineal in a strong way as there is more money in Viagra I suppose.

The amount of blood needed seems to show it had a more important job during ancient times and is E-M field receptors might have been used for all types of things. That being said, the amount of blood supplied shows us its importance and its similar eye structure tells us it is substantially associated with Bio-Photonics. Another thing we know is that Stress increases light output [perhaps as a plea!]. Stress seems to be very receptive to bio-photonic inputs.

Sleep Reset

Sleep may be required to reset the bio-photonic cycle. We know that Fluctuation in photon counts over the body is **lower in the morning** [after sleep] than in the afternoon. This seems to show the body is more stressed in the afternoon and may need to have reduced photon input to reduce stress. Additionally, studies show that the upper extremities and the head region emit most the bio-photonic emissions [not the hands] and the emissions increase over the day. [Something needs to halt the increase before problems arise.]

Without having some mechanism to reduce photon emissions, the brain could very well suffer as cell operation would be changed from <u>too much optical messaging.</u> One issue noted is that Multiple Sclerosis is identified as cells with <u>too many coherent biophotonic emissions</u>. Possibly, sleep allows the emissions to seek some level of disorder needed to provide us continued health. All that sounds interesting but just how do cells interact with received bio-photons from adjacent cells or the outside world? One inappropriate way is something called Free Radicals.

Free Radicals

It is well-known that all living organisms emit low intensity chemi-luminescence as part of their metabolic processes. When electrons move between energy states during chemical reactions as part of metabolic processes [Oxygenation of cells], photons are either be absorbed or emitted. A major source of photons is the breaking down of larger molecules into smaller ones resulting in the chemical byproducts of the reaction as well as emitted photons.

Recent research indicates that the presence of free radicals [reactive oxygen species and singlet oxygen] is associated with weakened immune function and various diseases. With more free oxygen to pair, more substantial chemi-luminescence is produced which we will investigate later. Sometimes the photonic messages are ok, but many times, the messages are flawed. They are either the wrong wavelength or too strong to initiate proper response. The cell goes into overdrive and sometime the wrong hydrocarbons read the wrong message initiating a runaway condition we call cancer.

Someone found that various vegetables would help flush the body of these free radicals and reduce the possibility of transmitting the wrong photonic message into the body. These vegetables may do even more. Let's take the old standard----Mistletoe. It may cure cancer.

Plant Cure of Cancer

Scientists around the globe studying the initiation and effect of bio-photons have begun to consider that your body's communication system might be a complex network of resonance and frequency. What if <u>vegetables actually changed the emissions of cells by combination and optical outputs like turning red light and green light into yellow light</u> or the stranger event of having red and blue photons combining to make <u>magenta?</u>

Magic Magenta

The only reason I brought up the last one is that **there is no magenta in nature** as blue and red are on separate sides of the rainbow. It is truly an oddball that has no wavelength on its own. What if adding fresh, <u>still radiating plants</u> into a person's body emitted signals that would combine with those aggressive outputs initiated by free radicals and the emissions together made a "color" that cancer cells simply could not understand? An advantage of this phenomenon is known as photo-repair. Let's see what happened with a <u>vegetable named mistletoe</u>. Here is what researcher Dr. Popp had to say again.

> *"If cancer-causing chemicals could alter the body's biophoton emissions, then it might be that other substances could reintroduce better communication. <u>Mistletoe appeared to help the body to 'resocialize'</u> the photon emissions of tumor cells back to normal.*

In one of numerous cases, Dr. Popp came across a woman in her thirties who had breast and vaginal cancer. He found <u>mistletoe</u> created something he called "coherence" in her cancer tissue samples. After a year, all her laboratory tests were virtually back to normal as the cancer had been "resocialized". Fresh mistletoe had transmitted photons into the body such that there was a direct or indirect modification of the cancer cell emissions.

> *He had found that <u>photonic messaging could cure cancer; so are there other vegetables that can help?</u>*

Fresh Fruits and Vegetables

Raw Organic Food

I am not one that pushes organic foods as there is no real way to determine how something was grown, but in Dr. Popp's experiments, he found that organic foods growing in the wild emitted twice as many biophotons as cultivated organic crops, and cultivated organics outputted substantially more than commercially grown foods. He also discovered that cooked or irradiated food emitted virtually no biophotons, so they are pretty much useless.

Freshly Picked

After wild plants, the next best source of biophotons are freshly picked, organically grown fruits and vegetables, according to Heinz R. Gisel, author of *"In Foodture We Trust."* He cites one study in which the bio-photonic radiation from fresh fruits and vegetables was compared with that from a multivitamin that contained all of the vitamins in the daily recommended amounts. While the radiation from the fresh foods was bright, that from the vitamins was <u>virtually nonexistent</u>. Yes, I think he was saying <u>those pills you take to make you healthy are pretty much rubbish</u>.

To get the highest level of biophotons, eat a diet rich in raw fruits and vegetables that have been freshly picked from your own organic garden. Alternatively, if live in the city with no garden and have no access to a family garden, head for the countryside and visit a farm where you can pick your own organically grown fruits and vegetables.

Plan on eating this produce as soon as possible after you get it if you want to reduce the chance of Cancer and other cell disruption type diseases. As the Photosynthesis deceases in picked plants so does the healing of those plants as their photosynthetic system begins to die.

Photosynthetic Messaging

Plants, cyanobacteria, and algae are all classed as oxygenic photosynthetic organisms. In these life forms, photons are absorbed by two large membrane protein complexes called Photosystem I [PS-I which absorbs mostly 700nm light], and Photosystem II [PS-II which absorbs mostly 670nm light]. Mostly this is done with special molecules called Chlorophylls. In these oxygen-producing organisms, carbon dioxide is "reduced" [electrons are added] to form sugars that the plant eats.

As mentioned chlorophylls absorb in the red and the blue spectral regions, reflect in the green as a useless color. This feature gives the green color to plant leaves. I shouldn't say it is completely useless as plants have something called phycocynin, which absorbs in the green and yellow region. The wide variety of photons turning carbon dioxide into oxygen not only make the food needed for the plants, but also retransmit optical messages as wavelength variations and optical pulsing to help control the plant's environment.

Inverted Bio-Photons

While animal cells convert energy from Oxygen and "free radicals", plants do the exact opposite to produce energy and Bio-photons. This is called photosynthesis. In photosynthesis, smaller molecules are combined with the absorption of photons from sunlight to create larger molecules. In humans, larger molecules are broken down to smaller ones to emit light.

While photosynthesis starts with light around 670 to 700nm, the optical messaging is a little different. From photosynthesis, low-level emissions from plants are related to chlorophyll and that the emissions have peaks in the vicinity of 400 nm [deep blue] as well as the regenerated 700 nm [deep red/infrared]. As the manufacture of the bio-photons is opposite to animal production, we can assume the wavelengths are substantially different in phasing, and polarization. We can believe the method for interface between plant and animal is in this difference. As different light colors, phases, pulsing, or polarizations come in contact, they make a different color with its own characteristics. Many times, it is the combined color message that is required for effective interface between cells. Without the raw vegetables, the color exchange can be disruptive or even malignant.

To a plant, that does not eat animals, it was believed the only communication link is by photosynthesis. Not only did this seem to be problematic in cell operation but also, the photosynthetic emissions were extremely weak so a plant could not affect plants nearby. That's where fungus comes in.

Fungus

Fungus expert Paul Stamets called them "*Earth's natural internet*" in a recent discussion of plant communications. In 2013 David Johnson of the University of Aberdeen and his colleagues showed that broad beans use fungal networks to pick up on impending threats – in this case, hungry aphids, but they are just as bad as disease to a human.

Johnson found that broad bean seedlings that were not themselves under attack by aphids, but were connected to those that were via fungal roots called mycelia, activated their anti-aphid chemical defenses so that fewer aphids attacked. This was not a smell transfer but an electromagnetic transfer. Bio-Photons generated codes that were channeled thought the cellular structure of the fungus to protect nearby plants.

We can think of it like laying one's hands on a sick person. In this case the sick lays his hands on the surrounding plants by using fungus. It seems that through these hands coded optical messages are transmitted.

Plant Messaging

Over the past couple of years researchers have observed patterns in the optical coding from plants. To researchers this messaging looks like patterns in the "optical noise" surrounding the plant parts. It appeared as if not only did the bio-photon patterns extended beyond the plants, but that patterns were strengthened between plants when they were in close proximity. It looks like simple transmission of continuous optical energy may not be what will allow us to understand how plants and animal cells talk, operate, get sick, and repair. "Technology Review" reported the following: *Biophotons from growing plants have been associated with increased cell division in other nearby plants at rates up to 30 percent.* By coding the messages, weak bio-photonic messages can be "seen" at fairly long distances. One thing that is being done to examine these messages is to look at fish eggs.

Fish Eggs

Bio-photonic communication between cells that are separated has a special name. Called the mito-genetic effect, this is the way cells can "somehow" have communications between distant samples [without fungus]. We know that bio-photons are produced at really low rates [a few dozen per second per square centimeter], but researcher Sergey Mayburov's began studying fish egg bio-photonic emission patterns. What he saw was a discernible structure in the stream of photons emanating from cellular bodies. Periodic bursts of biophotons resembled the patterns used to transmit binary data over noisy channels. To him, this explained how cells might be able to detect these extremely weak signals being transmitted across noisy environments.

"Technology Review" reported the following: *Biophotons from mature eggs have been shown to disrupt the growth of younger eggs. In some cases, this disruption seemed to stop the development of immature eggs entirely.*"

It was found that bio-photonic radiation performs the communications between distant samples, which resulted in the synchronization of egg development. The photon radiation in form of short quasi-periodic bursts was observed in both fish and frog eggs; hence the communication mechanism seems to be similar to the exchange of binary encoded data via the noisy channels. It was noted that the artificial constant illumination by the visible light, over 100 times more intense, could not induce the comparable gain. The communications of some other types were reported also; for the bio-systems in the state of abrupt stress or slow destruction [apoptosis] such radiation can change the state of other bio-systems in the similar depressive way. The question he tried to answer was if the stream of photons had any discernible structure that would qualify it as a form of communication, and the answer was-yes!

Eggs Synchronizing Eggs

Other experiments have shown that the biophotons from growing eggs can encourage the growth of other eggs of a similar age just like the biophotons from mature eggs hindered the growth of younger eggs at a different stage of development.

Long Distance Bio-Photons

According to Dr. Fritz Popp [again] *"Consciousness is responsible for a transformation process of potential information into current information"*. This means it is consciousness that collapses all the potential states of possibility in the quantum field to a specific physical reality. In this case <u>consciousness directly affects the transmission of bio-photons</u> or information packs required for our daily function.

Russian scientists have used bio-photon emission to measure communication between two entangled individuals at a distance. Dr. Konstantine Korotkov used what is called <u>Bio-Electrophotography</u> and observed how one individual can send a <u>telepathic message</u> that is instantly being received by another at a distance. I'm not sure about the method for transferring photon here, but Russians are really into such things.

Fish and Birds

Have you ever wondered how an entire school of fish can turn on a dime in the face of danger and how large groups of flying birds turn with prefect precision and never run into one another? It seems these, not well understood, phenomena may have to do with the instantaneous emission of bio-photonic messages travelling the speed of light to all the fish simultaneously so that biological functions can be synchronized without some fish yelling "time to turn". Maybe fish have an aura that can be sensed by adjacent fish, which is sensed by the next and next until all know to turn "Instinctively". If we want to do the same we need to increase our bio-photonic Aura.

Increasing Your Aura

I think it can be cautiously stated that if you enhance your capability to emit proper photonic message, your visible Aura would also be enhanced. The 3 main ways I understand that one can increase the aura associated with bio-photonic emissions is by "faith", Chi, and/or by eating the right, fresh vegetables. It may be that all three are needed simultaneously. Naturally grown fresh fruits and vegetables are rich in biophotons; that's obvious. You need not be a mystic who can see auras to understand. The reality of light waves, or bio-photon energy, is obvious and the concept that plant emissions somehow negate inappropriate or cancerous emissions seems also to be a reasonable premise. Chi and Faith may be somewhat more difficult to enhance as one must separate yourself from your-self and from the world. Somehow, this separation allows you to sense understand and build levels of Chi or faith needed to enable you to help others. In accomplishing this type of focus, your Aura would be enhanced.

In bio-photonics, quality and quantity are both keys to successful communication, treatment, and diagnosis. If we go back to Physicist Popp again briefly, he theorized that *"Biophoton light emissions of healthy people follow biological rhythms, and that those rhythms are connected to the measureable biorhythms of the earth. There is a direct correlation and an active resonance amidst land, food, and people.*" Ok; a lot of mumbo jumbo, but I think there is a nugget of truth in that being in tune with our natural surroundings rather than being stuck inside yourself is a key to gaining control over bio-photonic emissions.

Power of Positive Thinking

Certainly, you have heard this term. It seems that if you have positive thinking or "faith" you can affect those around you. I'm thinking if you begin to sense a bluish glow around someone, they have more control over their environment and the people around them by simply bio-photonic messaging. Some people have this level of control.

Some people can't even control their own bodily functions properly, but bio-photonic research is helping were other methods have not been successful. One such advance takes a simple blue light bulb. I'm told it's better than a little blue pill.

Erectile Dysfunction

Here is an unusual use of bio-photonics if you are drinking too much Fluorinated water of if you have another reason for the problem. In Basel, Switzerland they are studying a gene called [Eros] that reacts to blue light could offer a drug-free remedy for men with erectile dysfunction. Researchers there have tested something they call an erectile opto-genetic stimulator (EROS) gene placed in male rats. They found that it could be used to reliably "turn on" erections and in some cases cause ejaculation. It seems pretty complicated. When Eros was exposed to the light, a molecule called guanosine triphosphate changes to guanosine monophosphate which allows calcium channels to close. With a reduction in calcium, the muscles tense and blood flow increases in the erectile tissue.

No more need of the complex psychological factors to allow for a process to excite an organ, simply get near blue light. With an estimated 30 million American men affected by erectile dysfunction, according to the National Institutes of Health [About 4 percent of men in their 50s, 17 percent of men in their 60s, and 47 percent of men over 75 experience the condition.], blue lights are safer and easier than Viagra and other drugs. Another thing to notice is that with drugs, there still has to be response to stimulus and high blood pressure victims are discouraged from trying such things. All kidding aside, this is just one of the many remarkable bio-photonic advances that are being discovered every day. Below are images of a blue bulb and a string of blue LED lights. No telling what happens if someone changes all their light fixtures out to blue light.

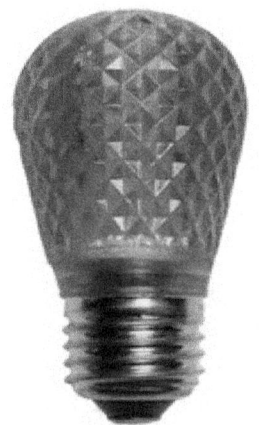 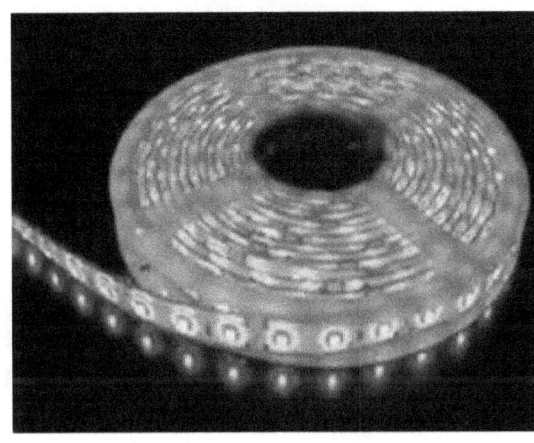

Don't make any jokes about Viagra being a blue pill or those blue tinted super bright headlights automobiles are using today and please do not look for blue condoms. It doesn't work like that. This is serious business. One question I have is, "Why women are always on Viagra commercials. Are they the only ones concerned about this problem?" While man doesn't typically shine brightly on his own, there are animals that do have visible halos and control them at will.

Bio-luminescence

This bio-photonics is a two-way process as photons may either be absorbed or emitted. A major source of photons being emitted is the breaking down of larger molecules into smaller ones resulting in the chemical byproducts of the reaction as well as emitted photons and that brings us to bio-luminescence. Within the field of bio-photonic there is a highly sensitive noninvasive, nontoxic technique based on the detection of visible light that arises from either the excitation of a fluorescent protein, molecule, or enzyme-catalyzed oxidation reaction. This is described by emission of light and is called bio-luminescence. Although the light emitted may be dim, it is detectable externally using sensitive photon detectors or intensified cameras mounted within light-tight specimen chambers. As light produced by this process passes through a range of tissue types, including skin, muscle and bone, researchers can observe and quantify the distribution of light production from within living animals which general tells the researcher the condition, disease, and metabolic processes of the area being viewed. Bioluminescence is the physical glow of animals, bacteria, etc. It is widely distributed in nature, occurring in a remarkably diverse set of organisms, including bacteria, fungi, fish, insects, shrimp and squid. Yanking out the luminance production mixtures is very useful in investigations in animal injury and disease tracking and treating by making proteins or minerals fluoresce. Bioluminescence arises from the oxidation of a substrate called a luciferin by an enzyme called a luciferase, which usually requires energy and oxygen. Luciferin and luciferase are simply generic terms so don't get too bogged down with them. There are five basic luciferin–luciferase/Bio-luminance systems. Most widely studied of the bioluminescence systems are those belonging to luminous beetles in the family Lampyridae [fireflies, click beetles, the sea pansy, the marine copepod and a wide variety of luminous bacteria, so let's see how this bioluminescence form of photon emission can help us.

Squid and cuttlefish are exceptional in how they can use this luminescence to hypnotize victims and convert their skin color to look exactly like the background in a split second. Next is an example of one of the luminous creatures in and out of the light.

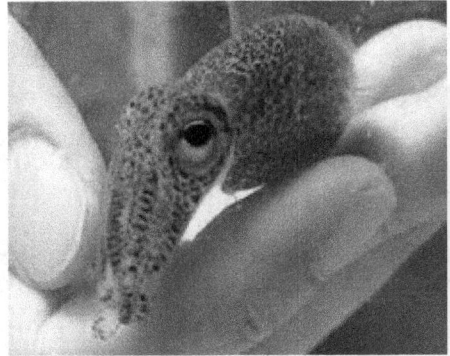 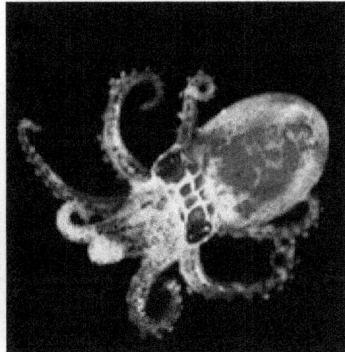

Beetles

The beetle luminescence reaction is catalyzed by a luciferase oxidizing luciferin resulting in the production of oxyluciferin, CO_2, and the emission of light. That has a peak wavelength of 560 nm with light peaks, ranging from 546 to 593 nm. Sometimes these distinct frequencies are needed, but the firefly luminance oxyluciferin is used more often in animal studies. Below is one such beetle. To the right the beetle is now glowing bright yellow for whatever he wanted that color for.

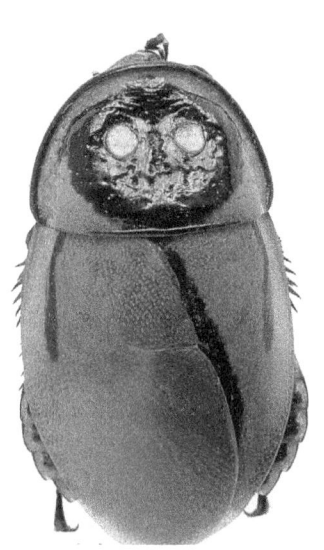 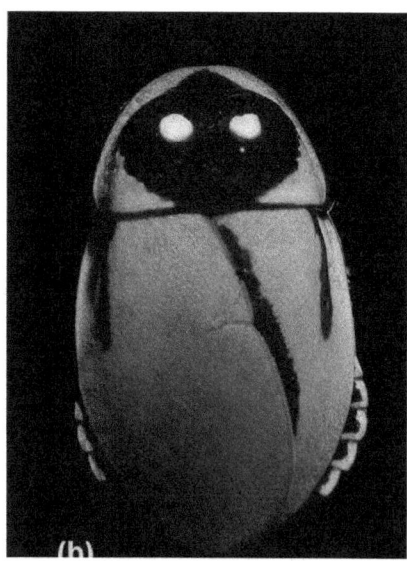

Firefly

The light generated by the firefly luciferase is influenced by temperature, shifting to a peak of 610 nm at 37 °C. The firefly luciferase catalyzes <u>the most efficient bioluminescent reaction</u> known. [The amount of light generated in relation to the energy expended is extremely low.] Therefore, it is the one normally used for treatment and research. Next are the firefly and glow worm that are very common contributors to this science.

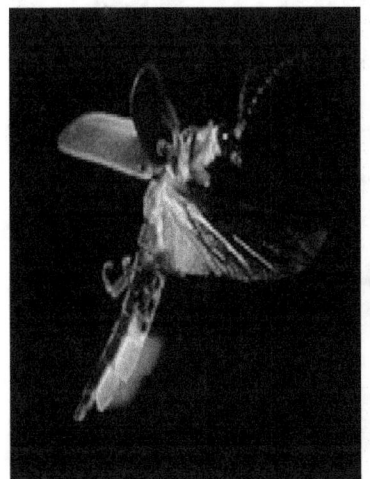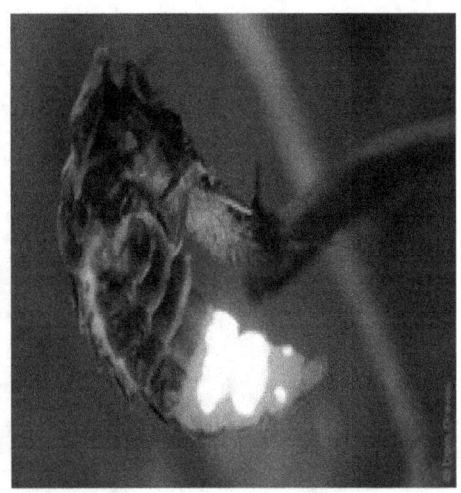

Mouse Tumors

To experiment on mice, luciferin must be administered by an appropriate route, most commonly via intraperitoneal injection, a few minutes before imaging. Fortunately, at the doses administered, luciferin does not kill the animals and rapidly distributes throughout the mouse, crossing the blood–brain, placental barriers or direct view of muscles, joints, the vaginal tract, the nasal and pulmonary airways or within food and water before luminescence studies allow details of disease, and issue to show up for Bio-photonic inspections. The set of images below tracks the luminescent material to areas of wound or disease.

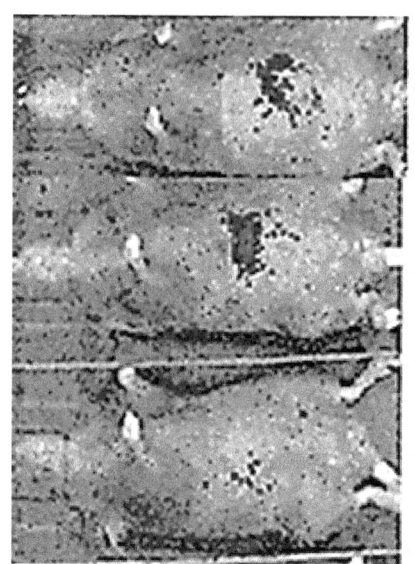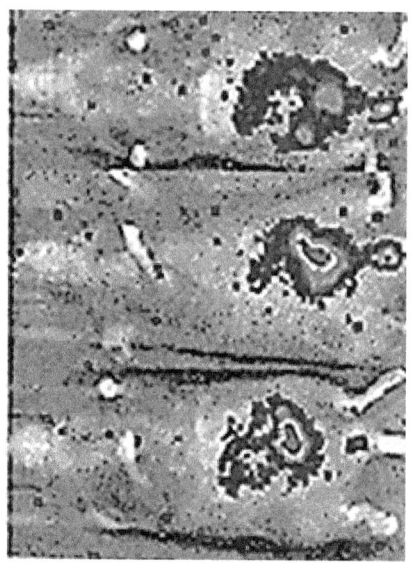

Sea Pansy

The sea pansy and copepod luciferases, are developed by genes called *rluc* and *gluc*. *These are* considered the most common natural bio-luminescence system, especially for deep-sea animals. So far, they believe there are seven distinct phyla and approximately 90 genera. In this case the gene Coelenterazine that is oxidized by the appropriate luciferase to carbon dioxide and light in the blue part of the spectrum [480 nm]. Interestingly, this stuff has been found in mammalian and bacteria cells as well. This coelenterazine stuff is highly chemi-luminescent, so it is somewhat easier to use when reactions are subtle. As shown below left under "normal" lighting, the sea pansy looks like a normal animal, but in the dark, it shines bright blue and shown to the right.

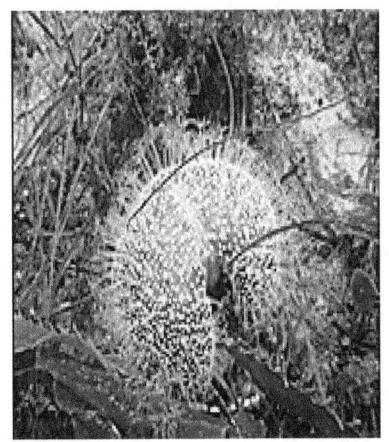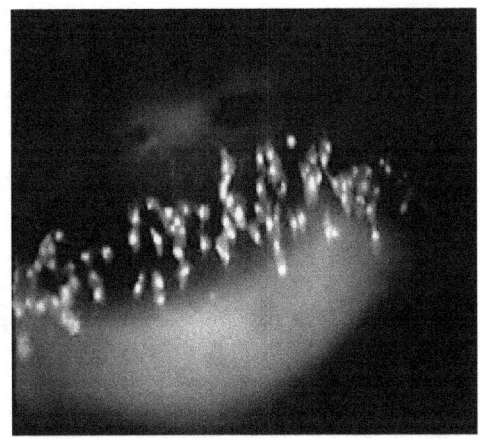

Bacterial Luminescence

The bacterial luminescence reaction involves the oxidation of an aldehyde that is reduced by Flavin to form Oxi-flavin and light at 490 nm which has other special effects on cells. The images show some of these special bacteria that are being used to find and treat disease.

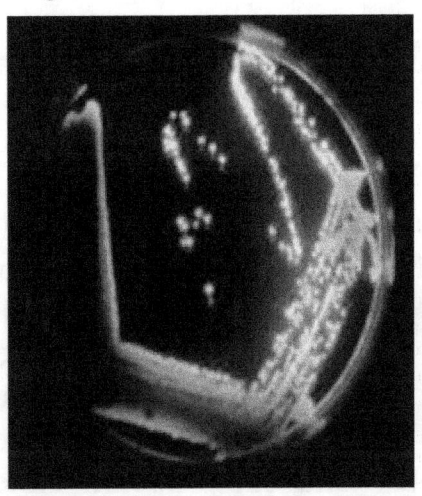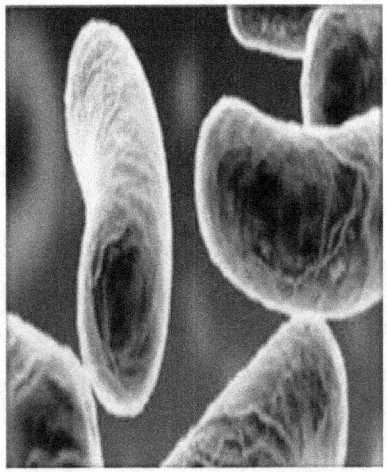

Fluorescence

The phenomenon of fluorescence was first described in 1845 by John Frederick William Herschel, who observed a superficial blue glow in a solution of quinine in the sunlight. The intervening years have now seen Fluorescent probes used all the time in biological research. Irradiation of a fluorescent compound with light of a suitable wavelength leads to the transition of an electron in the molecule to a higher energy state called <u>excitation</u>. This process is almost instantaneous. Upon return of the electron to a lower energy level, <u>light of lower energy is emitted, giving the fluorescent signal</u>. Because lower energy light is emitted, it is <u>red-shifted</u> in the spectrum when compared with the excitation light, a phenomenon known as the Stokes shift.

Stokes Shift

In general, anything losing energy changes its wavelength by becoming redder. The following graph shows how various important tissues that fluoresce change wavelength as a Stokes Shift. Notice how they emit at a much redder [longer wavelength]. The graph starts in the UV region and shows wavelengths almost to visible red. As an example, Tryptophan absorbs 230nm UV and emits 350nm violet light.

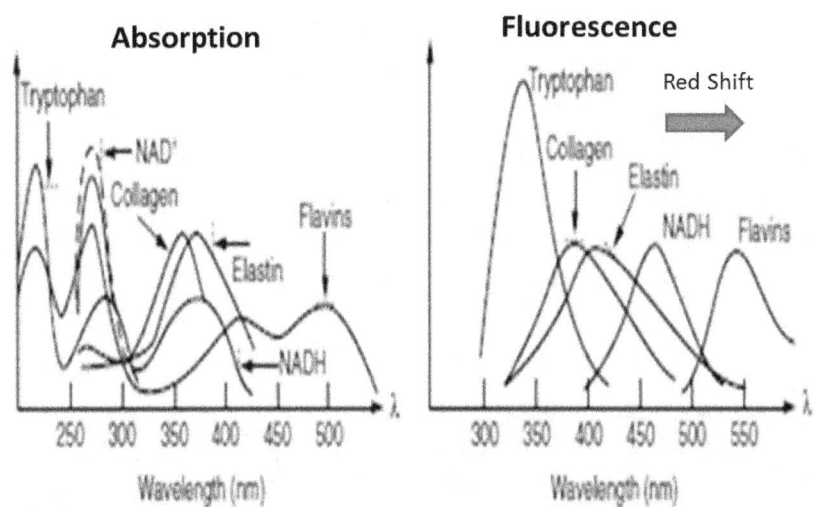

Additional Fluorescence materials are shown below which allow for up to deep red emission.

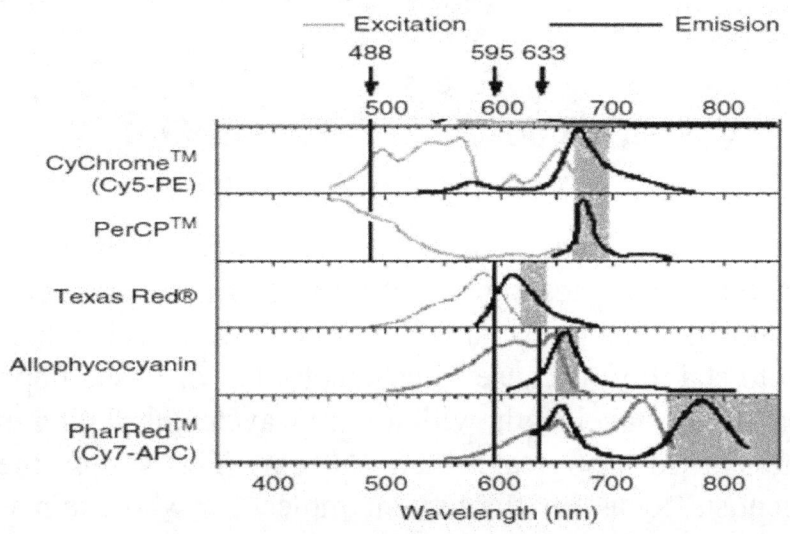

Jelly Fish

Green <u>fluorescent protein [FP]</u> from the jelly fish *Aequorea victoria* was first described in 1962 by Osamu Shimomura who was awarded the <u>2009 Nobel Prize in Chemistry</u> for his discovery. In the last 15 years scientist have found or artificially developed numerous FPs in all colors of the rainbow have been discovered and developed. Cyan to chromo-red colored Fluorescent Proteins [FPs] are often based on proteins from sea organisms such as coral. As these materials are introduced, they convert photons into different colors that can be examined for a wide variety of issues. A couple of corals exhibiting these FPs are shown below. These fluoresce in the green and blue-green region.

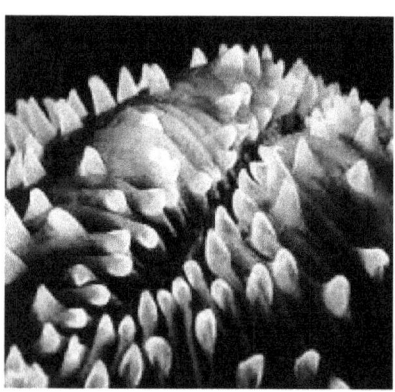 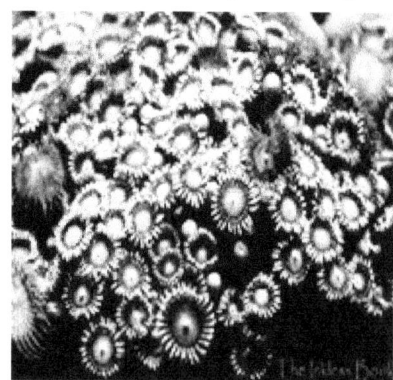

Visibility Through Cells

For a fluorescent marker to be successfully used in treatment and testing it has to fulfil several criteria including suitable excitation and emission wavelengths and photo-stability, because light penetration of tissue depends heavily on wavelength, with longer wavelengths being more efficient [ideally greater than 650 nm]. This simply means scientists focus on fluorescent molecules whose emission are in the red or the far-red end of the spectrum, which are most suitable for penetrating into and through cells for inspection.

As cells are mostly made of water transmission through them means we must transmit through water. Luckily, water does not have any absorption bands from UV to near IR. It starts absorbing weakly above 1.3um, with more pronounced peaks at wavelengths 2.9um and very strong absorption at 10um, the wavelength of a CO_2 laser beam. Therefore, most cells exhibit very good transparency between 0.8um and 3um. Wow! It is like whoever created us thought that seeing through our cells would be an important thing or he wanted the body to run on photonic emission and fluorescence.

CRP Fluorescence

Some materials in our bodies fluoresce on their own. One such protein is C-reactive protein [CRP] in serum. CRP determination can be extremely important for physicians to define the etiology of sepsis. The circulating concentration of human CRP in healthy patients is about 5 mg per liter. In the presence of infection, these values can raise up to about 500 mg per liter. As the general graph next shows, as infection gets worse, emitted CRP fluorescence increases. You tell your doctor you don't feel right, He checks the fluorescence of your body through the water in your cells and confirms your analysis.

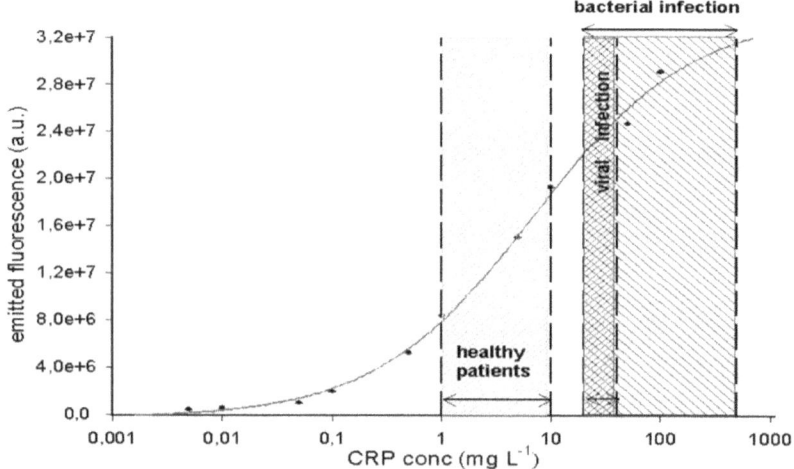

The next graph shows how a breast can be irradiated with 488nm emissions and its fluorescence can determine if a tumor is present well before self-examination can make that determination.

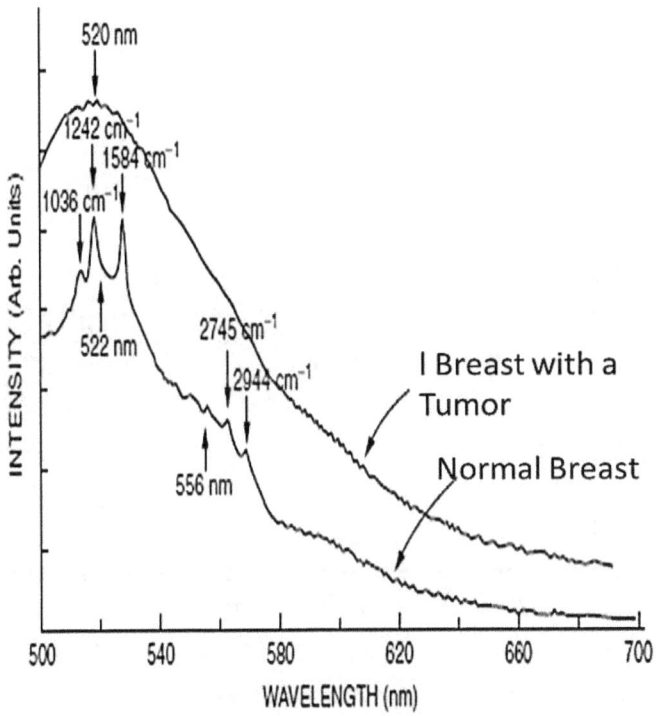

All this is nice but just finding cancer with photonic signal is one thing. We need to eliminate bad cells.

Photodynamic Elimination

From all of this, photodynamic therapy (PDT) has emerged as a promising treatment of cancer and other diseases utilizing activation of an external chemical agent, called a photosensitizer or PDT drug, by light. This drug is administered either intravenously or topically to the malignant site as in the case of certain skin cancers. Then light of a specific wavelength, which can be absorbed by the PDT photosensitizer, is applied. The PDT drug absorbs this light, <u>producing reactive oxygen species that can destroy the tumor.</u>

This type of process induced by a photosensitizer initially has been showing great promise for cancers, but the list is now growing concerning what researchers believe will be an ACTUAL treatment of deadly disease.

Potential Treatments

The following list describes some of the initial experimental treatments being tried by this bio-photonic process.

- Micro invasive non-small-cell lung cancer
- Other lung tumors
- Cancer of the esophagus

- Early-stage esophageal cancer
- Skin cancers
- Breast cancer
- Brain tumors
- Colorectal tumors
- Gynecologic malignancies
- Alternative to angioplasty
- Chronic skin diseases
- Rheumatoid arthritis
- Macular degeneration
- Wound healing, oral cavity
- Antiviral
- Anticancer Vaccines
- Endometriosis

Even when this is not a possibility, there is new research locating cancerous cells using bio-photonics that also looks like it will save lives.

Cancer Blasting

A brand new, combined imaging and phototherapy technique may guide surgeons removing chemotherapy-resistant tumors and kill any cancer cells the surgeons miss, so we had better look at this as well. Experiments with mice have showed remarkable success of locating ALL cancer for blasting in ovarian cancer infected mice. To top it off, the mice showed no apparent side effects or weight loss following the procedure. As my daughter died of this horrible disease, this is of special interest. To do this, special micro-particles were designed to carry drugs. The compound name is <u>silicon naphthalocyanine</u>. Like many of these bio-photonic treatment ideas, this stuff fluoresces when exposed to near-infrared light [785nm] and it loves cancer cells. In addition to highlighting cancerous tissue, the drug also generates cancer-killing reactive oxygen species when illuminated so one gets internal blasting directed only at the cancer in addition to showing where to blast the remaining cancer.

Increasing Blood Flow

A team led by Johns Hopkins Medicine discovered the receptor, which causes blood vessels to relax in response to bio-photonics. Even more interesting, it was found that blood vessel function can be regulated through changing light wavelengths.

Blood Eyes

This is when they really gained some bio-photonic insight as it was determined that blood seems to "see" the light as it contains something called Melanopsin. Melanopsin is a type of photo-pigment belonging to a larger family of light-sensitive retinal proteins [or Opsins]. When researchers found blood with this Opsin, the vessels would relax in response to light. Once relaxed, one could enhance blood flow. Tested on a restricted mouse tail showed positive results that will, hopefully, allow for reasonable bio-photonic treatment of something called Raynaud's phenomenon, which is characterized by exaggerated vasoconstriction of the vessels of the fingers and toes, which is probably just as horrible as is sounds. As shown below, the left image of blood flow shows almost no entry while the lower hand looks reasonable. The effect is death to parts of the fingers and toes as shown to the right.

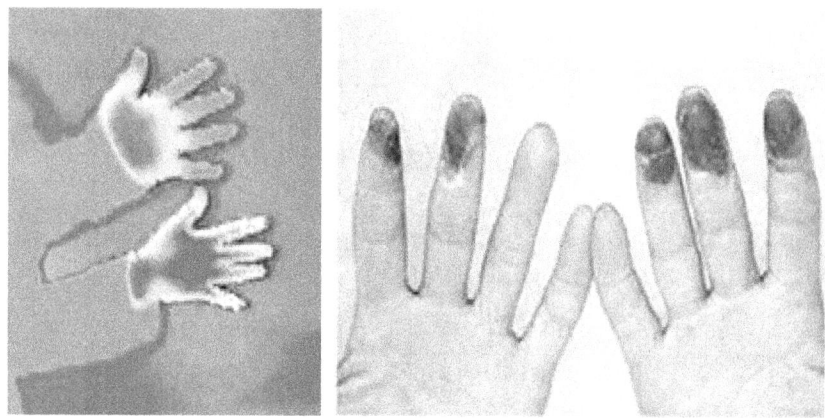

The next step is to use high-intensity LEDs incorporated into gloves and socks as a potential mode of therapy for these patients. While somewhat different in concept, these studies sound similar to others be looked at for faster diabetic healing.

Faster Diabetic Healing

This is very important Bio-photonic research focusing on increasing the life of diabetic patients by allowing their bodies to heal. Low-energy laser irradiance at certain wavelengths is able to stimulate the tissue bio-reaction and enhance the healing process. This is especially important when diabetes restricts new growth so drastically. Collagen deposition is one of the important aspects in healing process because it can also increase the strength of the skin. It seems that biphotonic irradiation increases collagen production needed for diabetic wounds in rats. The tensile strength of skin was employed as a parameter to describe the wound. The number of cases of diabetes mellitus (DM) worldwide is estimated to be around 150 million. This is predicted to *double by 2025* with the greatest number of cases in China and India. Diabetic foot and leg ulcer (DFU or DLU) is a serious complication of DM and is the single most important risk factor for lower limb amputations. More than 60% of all non-traumatic lower limb amputations are due to DFU complications. To make that even worse, around 50% of all non-traumatic amputations are as a result of DM. To further highlight the seriousness of diabetes associated lower-limb amputations, the 5-year mortality rate following amputation stands at 40 to 80%. Foot and leg ulcers are serious complications of Diabetes Mellitus (DM) and are known to be resistant to conventional treatment. They may herald severe complications if not treated wisely. That's where bio-photonics comes in. Electromagnetic radiations in the form of photons are delivered to the ulcers to stimulate healing. This first study was conducted to evaluate the efficacy of Low-Level-Laser-Therapy (LLLT) in diabetic ulcer healing dynamics. Once the photon energy is absorbed, the photo acceptor assumes an electronically excited state. One idea is that this stimulates cellular metabolism by activating or deactivating enzymes which can alter DNA and RNA. The energy which is absorbed by the photo acceptor can be transferred to other molecules giving us observable effects at a biological level. Photon energy is absorbed by cells, which activates secondary messengers and cascades the healing optical code.

Diabetic Rats

In one important experiment, diabetic wounded rats had large wounds induced by streptozotocin via intravenous injection. Skin-breaking strength was measured using an Instron tensile test machine. The experimental animals were treated with bio-photonic emissions at 808nm using a diode laser. The photo-stimulation effect was revealed by accelerated healing process and enhanced tensile strength of wound. Laser photo-stimulation on tensile strength in diabetic wound suggests that such therapy facilitates collagen production in diabetic wound healing which will soon reduce suffering of diabetic patients.

LED Therapy

Besides these laser tests, lower intensity RED LED emissions have successfully been used to halt and reverse effects of this horrible life stressing condition. The following image shows one of the LED emission tools used for this type of Therapy

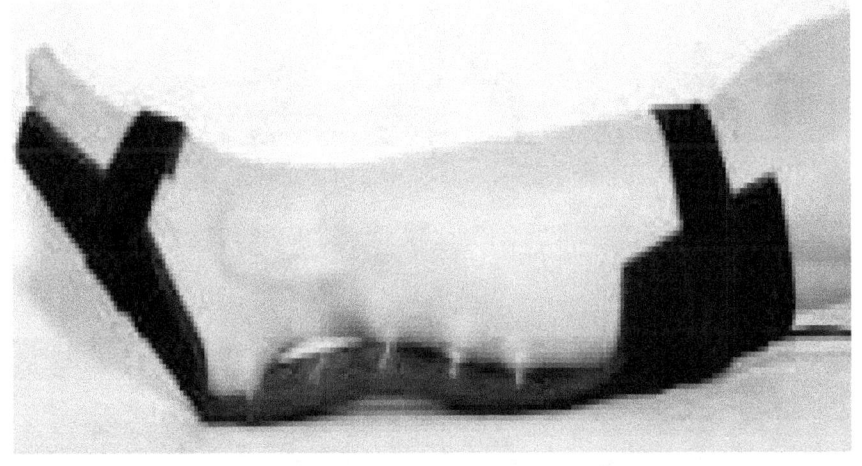

The diabetic ulsers on feet and legs are being removed by 670nm red light almost like the 808nm Laser light.

The next images show just how effective and rapid this type of theraphy is and no cutting off of legs and long hospital stays and loss of life savings. The firse image was of a diabetic patient almost ready for amputation as the leg was in terrible shape. The following shows a typical diabetic leg ulser treated over a 4 month time with "light". The ulcers almost seem to disappear before our very eyes as cells are messaged to change from a dying state to a rejouvenation state. Its like magic or laying on of hands. [Sorry for the nasty pictures, but these are so much less nasty than many of the horrors associated with diabetes so get over complaining.]

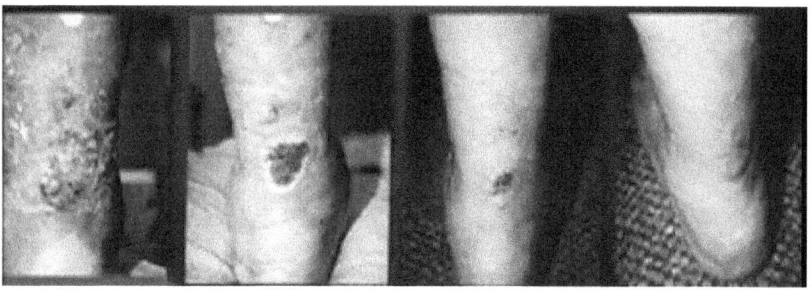

Optical Glucose Sensing

If you are diabetic, you know that you need to continuously check your blood. Current methods are totally chemical based, but there is good research converting this tedious prick your finger method into a bio-photonic method that will hopefully, make it much easier, make the interfaces reusable and possibly even provide continuous checking for immediate recognition of any problem.

The measurement of glucose is among the most important analytical tasks. It has been estimated that about 40% of all blood tests are related to it so we are not just limited to diabetes here. In addition, there are numerous other situations where glucose is to be determined, for example, in biotechnology, the production and processing of all kinds of food, in biochemistry in general, and in numerous other areas. The continuing interest in sensing glucose, mainly in blood, is one result of the increasing age the world's population, and the fact that about 4% of its Caucasian population suffers from diabetes.

The market for glucose sensors is probably the biggest single one in the diagnostic field, its size being about <u>$40 billion per year at present</u>. Given this size, it does not come as a surprise that any true improvement in sensing glucose represents a major step forward. The greatest need at present is, however, for continuous sensors.

Pacemaker Testing-Besides diabetics, scientists are looking at elimination of electrodes for patients with heart pacemakers.

Oxygen Testing- A couple of reversible optical sensors rely on the measurement of the consumption of oxygen. Among the optical methods, photometry, fluorescence, and something called surface plasmon resonance (SPR) are beginning to find success.

Special Contact lenses- One thought was to coat lenses with special materials that would change color if inappropriate materials pass by the lens.

If you see someone with red eyes, they may not be werewolves. I would stay as far away as I could just in case, but the testing sounds interesting.

Special Bandages- Another way to provide continuous optical testing of the blood might be Band-Aids.

Phosphorescent Bandage

One more bio-photonic trick being used in labs is a way to look at oxygenation of wounds like diabetic ulcers through special bandages. What about a "smart" bandage that can indicate oxygen concentration in severely damaged tissue? This invention increases the success rate of surgeries to restore limbs and physical functions by allowing visual indication of oxygenation without having to remove bandages. These special bio-photonic things are see-through, paint-on bandages providing "almost" direct, noninvasive measurement of tissue oxygenation using an imaging method that captures oxygen-dependent signals from the bandage.

This bandage was made with an oxygen-sensitive phosphor and a green oxygen-insensitive reference dye to clearly demonstrate the changes in tissue oxygenation. It was painted onto the skin as a viscous liquid, which dried into a solid film in less than a minute. A second barrier layer was then applied to protect the film and slow the rate of oxygen exchange between the bandage and the air.

All that was needed then was an electronic flash at 400nm [blue]. The phosphor activates around the near-infrared spectrum that is less excited with more oxygen. The variations in color also allow for detailed understanding of oxygenation. While this may help us quickly understand where and when there are differences in the blood, the brain may take a little different tact.

Brain Label

Speaking of new uses for Bio-photonics, in Ashburn, Virginia, researchers have just designed a new optical labeling method they called CaMPARI, [Calcium-modulated, photoactivatable, ratiometric integrator]. I know it a mouthful or a brain-full, but the idea is to build a marker that would fluoresce in a drastically different color [bright pink] than the background [violet light] when calcium molecules were sense in while in a bath of light. To stop the reaction, the light is turned off. So far, successful treatments of fruit-flies, Zebra-fish, and mice all have allowed immediate, on the fly, moving diagnostics of brain function that completely corresponds to much more tedious data taken by non-bio-photonic means. The material frees scientists from the need to use a microscope to observe neuronal activity. The label has been tested in living mice, fruit flies and zebra-fish. No longer does the animal have to be under a microscope during an experiment so reaction information can be accumulated much faster, easier, and more effectively than predecessor testing. I know some of you are wondering if they get blue and violet lamps mixed up, but let's go on.

Photonic Brain Manipulation

Our brains typically stay in states called Alpha, beta and Gamma which mean the main Vibrational characteristic of a brain [not in coherence] is between 8 and 100 hertz as shown in the following chart. When the brain senses coherence with the Heart-brain, it slows down substantially. What is interesting is that if one can slow down the rhythmic nature of the heart, all types of things begin to happen. The brain can be manipulated by very low frequency electro-magnetic messaging and by high frequency E-M waves. The following details are broken down by wavelength and "Common Name".

Epsilon Emissions <0.5Hz

- Extraordinary and Ecstatic states of consciousness
- High states of meditation and inspiration states
- Out-of-body experiences and Suspended animation

Delta Emissions   0.2 to 4 Hz

- Slow wave and Deep sleep with Lucid dreaming
- Confusion or disorientation with intuition
- Increased immune functions Miracle type healing,
- Hypnosis, Trance, and Near-death experience
- Blissful Inner being and personal growth,
- Trauma recovery and even Anti-aging

Theta Emissions   4 – 7 Hz

- Deep relaxation, meditation, and inner peace

- Increased memory, focus, and reduced mental fatigue
- Recall, and clear subconscious images .and creativity
- Physical and emotional healing
- Lower blood pressure
- Twilight sleep learning, wisdom, and Faith
- Sexual arousal and Vivid mental imagery
- Remote viewing and enhanced psychic abilities

Alpha Emissions   8 – 12 Hz

- Light relaxation with pleasant drifting feelings
- Positive thinking and creative problem solving
- Elevated mood and stress reduction
- Intuitive insights, Daydreams, and Calmness

Beta Emissions   12 – 30 Hz

- Anxious thinking and Arousal and alertness
- Analytical problem solving,
- Judgment, Decision making
- Increased mental ability, Focus, and concentration
- Good for absorbing information passively,
- Treating Hyperactivity and sensorimotor rhythm
- Outer awareness, survival, and dendrite growth

Gamma Emissions   30 – 100 + Hz

- Motor and cognitive functions heightened
- Advanced learning ability and boosted memory
- Enhanced perception of reality and compassion
- Binding of all senses: sight, smell, touch
- High-level information processing and energy levels
- Natural antidepressant, Positive thoughts
- Muscle development and release of growth hormone
- Recover from injuries and rejuvenation effects

Let me just give you a few of the frequencies in case you want to try some of this stuff.

Hertz	Condition
0.30	Depressions
0.40	Confusion
0.50	Relaxing
0.90	Euphoria
1.00	Feeling of well-being
3.50	Feeling of unity
3.60	Remedy for anger
5.80	Reduced Fear
6.26	Confusion
6.30	Accelerated learning
7.83	Stress tolerance
8.6	Induced sleep
15.0	Euphoria

While the military is experimenting with broadcasting subsonic waves to affect brainwaves and enhance the Delta levels [to confuse and put fear in an enemy], many are now trying to tap into meditative states and learning ability by transmitting the 40 Hertz level. What we are finding is that simple stereo speakers may be the best tool to introduce these enhancers. A 200-hertz tone is shot into one ear and a 200-hertz [plus the desired subsonic frequency] sound is transmitted into the other ear. The brain gets both of these frequencies and tries to mix them together to understand the sound. When the 2 frequencies a beat together, the output becomes the difference or only the subsonic vibrations are established as E-M field intrusions. Please notice the following:

Epsilon Thinking-If the brain is operating below about ½ Hertz people sense out-of-body experiences, spiritual insight, high levels of inspiration, and a high state of meditations. Introduction of this type of signal has been shown to force the brain into this level of activation.

Delta Thinking- [Less than 4 Hertz] produces a hypnotic state and also has an increase in intuition as well as some healing from trauma.

Theta Thinking [less than 7 hertz] increases memory function, increases creativity, gives a profound inner peace with emotional healing, and allows for psychic imagery.

While the heart does this simply by sending the Coherence massages, researchers are now simulating the heart with external devices. Because they have to get through bone, the signals must be stronger, but the idea is to force the brain into a lower state and bones will be repaired, stress will be eliminated, and on and on. Here is the interesting part. Test labs across the country are affecting our bodies simply by changing our brain base frequencies and watching in amazement sort of like when you watch a "faith healer". It seems completely bogus, but there you have a cured person. Just image how amazed the people were when one of the disciples would simply touch them and they could see, or stand, or whatever, and they did it without a machine.

Sphincter Resonance-The various successes are described below but first, we must talk about a failure. This can be illustrated with something called Sphincter Resonance about 4 Hz. In the 1960s, somebody supposedly discovered the resonating frequency of the sphincter. Presumably, this team created a device called an "Anal Sphincter Resonator". It was supposedly kind of like a musical organ. The idea was to intensify the suspense in movies whenever "Danger" was about to be portrayed. BACKFIRE and more BACKFIRE. Apparently, it caused the entire audience to soil themselves. The specific group of tones generated by this contraption has been referred to as a 'Brown Note' for some reason that I am not going into at this time. The specific notes have been lost over time, so I'm sure one of these mishaps will occur again in the future. This brings us to something very useful as scientist have found ways to introduce low frequency emissions directly into the brain by some interesting methods.

Brain Communications-Generally speaking brain control seems to require extremely low E-M field emissions to re-align neurons properly. While the shock treatment as such used decaying resonators to establish low wavelengths on the order of 100 Hz or so, we are now talking about much lower than that. The report *"A Review of Published Research on Low Frequency Noise and its Effects"* contains a long list of research about exposure to high-level infrasound among humans and animals. For instance, in 1972, Borredon exposed 42 young men to tones at 7.5 Hz at 130 dB for 50 minutes. While tones are not the same as E-M fields, we soon find that the response is from a manufactured E-M field rather than reception of these very low sub-audio signals.

In 1975, Slarve and Johnson exposed four male subjects to infrasound at frequencies from 1 to 20 Hz, for eight minutes at a time, at levels up to 144 dB SPL. There was no evidence of any detrimental effect other than middle ear discomfort. Tests of high-intensity infrasound on animals resulted in measurable changes, such as cell changes and ruptured blood vessel walls. Anytime someone says cell changes I'm thinking Cancer.

Making these ultralow subsonic E-M radiations was almost impossible in the free air so various machines were created. The Infratonic Qui Gong Machine, for instance, was developed out of scientific research in Beijing China which studied natural healers and found that most powerful "healers" were able to emit a strong infrasonic (low frequency) signals from their hands. While others did this type of emission, average individuals were only a hundredth as strong. The "Infratonic" brain/Neuron modification, is now used by 1% of all doctors in the United States. The images below show the Qui Gong and the Keely machine. Both provide these ultra-low subsonic emissions. A Dr. Keely designed relied on straight electro-magnetic fields being generated in a helmet of sorts. I don't know how successful this machine was, but it illustrates the point that everyone is trying to artificially excite different levels of consciousness and some are beginning to get success.

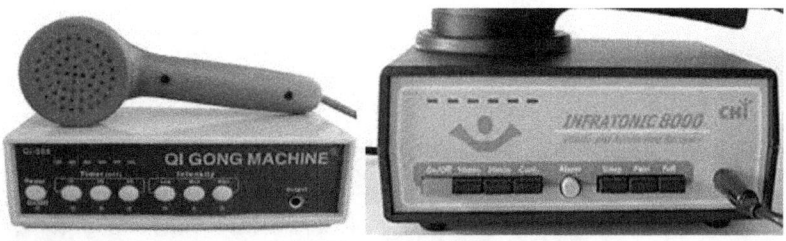

Today, there is a more portable system that is gaining acceptance. By sending in music in one ear and the same music [very slightly slower] in the other ear, the difference E-M field is generated and the neuron cells are excited just the same. Because the audio signals are much higher frequency, they can be generated in standard earphones as shown below.

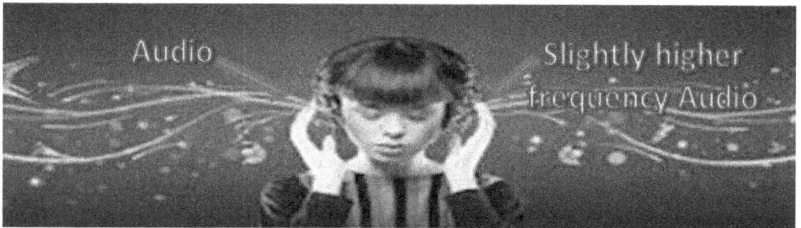

This method is called binaural interpretation as the actual subsonic modulation is not made by the emitter. Instead the difference frequency between the signals form each ear makes a combined signal that is subsonic and allows the brain to be communicated with to help in its repair in some way. Another way is to use moving magnets to build the E-M signals directly.

Transcranial Magnetic Stimulation (TMS)

Dr. Keely designed something called the 'Krell Helmet' back in the 1960s that relied on electro-magnetic fields generated in the helmet to cause modifications of brain activity and capability. I don't know how successful this machine was, but it would be the beginnings of something called Transcranial Magnetic Stimulation [TMS]. Rather than having a massive transmitter, this uses a massive pulsing magnet that is passed across the brain at a very slow rate which modulated an E-M field at subsonic rates similar to the Heart Brain. Today you can find these things everywhere, John Hopkins, the Mayo Clinic, and on and on we can go. In the early days, modulations needed to message the brain were done manually. Today, rather than having to physically pass a magnet across the brain, machines move the fields around to do all sorts of things for the brain. For those remembering the old TVs, it's like degaussing the brain, and has a similar effect to the degaussing coils that were modulated in the large CRT tube to stabilize the electric fields, and possibly that is what the Heart messaging does to send messages to regulate the body from time to time.

TMS is defined as a non-invasive method of brain stimulation that relies on electromagnetic induction using an insulated coil placed over the scalp. Sometimes it is focused on an area of the brain thought to play a role in mood regulation and other times it is moves around larger areas. The coil generates brief magnetic pulses. The pulse rates are kept secret, but we can imagine they are less than a couple of Hertz. The pulses are of extreme levels similar to an MRI machine, just to get though the scalp and into the brain, The Heart doesn't have to go through a skull so its job is easier. Here is the thing, these external Heart-message-simulators are producing fantastic results with lasting reductions in pain, and emotional stress without the side effects of drugs. The devices shown below are similar of those used at doctor's offices. Notice the last one is a handheld manual one. There are many, many types and sizes of these things being used today and most don't even know they are simulating the Heart-brain.

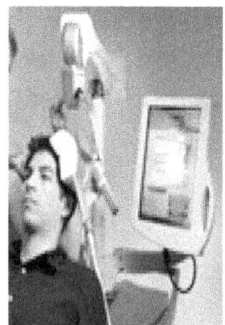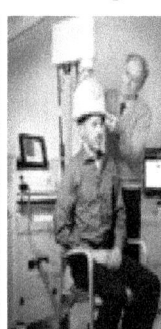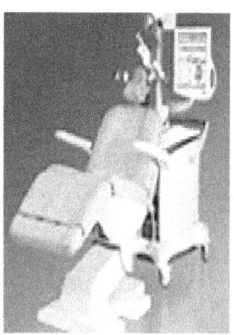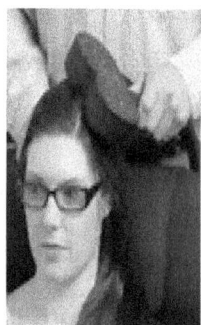

Interestingly this was first used on Rats and it was found that they not only healed wounds faster, but that they were able to learn how to trace mazes faster. The rats got smarter. I would say the Rats got wiser, but then I would sound like one of those Biblical writers describing the Heart.

Anti-Depression Communications-Let's talk about depression some more. If you are suffering from depression, you are not alone.

Approximately 16 million people in the U.S. live with this serious illness, but worse than that; about 4 million of these do not benefit from standard antidepressant medication

Electroconvulsive therapy [ECT], first developed in the 1940s, for years had a poor reputation with many negative depictions in popular culture. [See the image below left and then remove it from your mind.] Electro-Shock therapy showed up in many horror films as a way of destroying someone's brain or personality. However, the procedure has improved significantly since its initial use and is safe and effective. It uses a very high voltage of a low frequency E-M emission to re-associate the brain function. While over 100 thousand patients get this treatment every year, we still don't know exactly what happens.

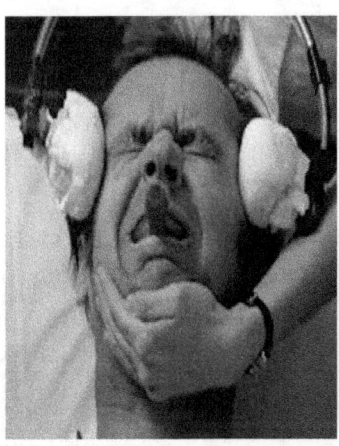 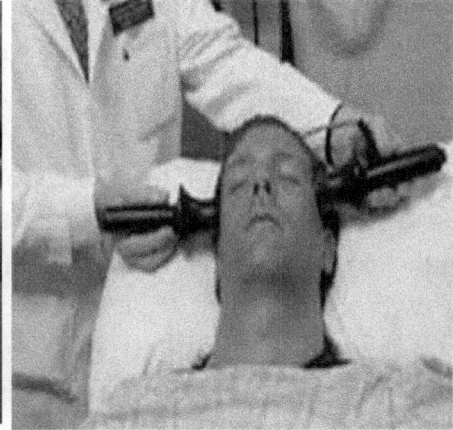

People who undergo ECT do not feel any pain or discomfort during the procedure. [See the previous image to the right of the one I told you to ignore.]

ECT is usually considered only after a patient's illness has not improved after other treatment options, such as antidepressant medication or psychotherapy, are tried. It is most often used to treat severe, treatment-resistant depression, but occasionally it is used to treat other mental disorders, such as bipolar disorder or schizophrenia. It also may be used in life-threatening circumstances, such as when a patient is catatonic, is suicidal, or is malnourished as a result of severe depression. One study, the Consortium for Research in ECT study, found an 86 percent remission rate for those with severe major depression. The same study found it to be effective in reducing chances of relapse when the patients underwent follow-up treatments.

While scientists are unsure how the treatment works to relieve depression, it appears to produce many changes in the chemistry and functioning of the brain. They also now know that usually 12 treatments are needed for reasonable long-term results. One possible clue to how the brain is affected is that people have a little trouble remembering information learned shortly after the procedure, but this difficulty usually disappears over the days and weeks following the end of an ECT course. It is possible that a person may have gaps in memory over the weeks during which he or she receives treatment. In the past, a "low level sine-wave" was used to administer electricity in a constant, high dose.   [Much of the Electrical burst was not modulated. Today, they use pulses which modulates the entire electrical pulse.

 If you are hugely sick, another E-M field treatment seems to be more appropriate it is called Repetitive transcranial magnetic stimulation. Like the method described above, E-

M fields penetrate cells to activate DNA emissions in various ways. By modifying the frequency, amplitude, cells irradiated, and sequence of modulation, each of these methods have different results so we are looking at each separately.

Repetitive Transcranial Magnetic Stimulation

Repetitive transcranial magnetic stimulation (rTMS) uses a moving magnet instead of an electrical current to activate the brain. The motion of the magnet causes a very low frequency E-M field modulation. First developed in 1985, rTMS has been studied as a possible treatment for depression, psychosis, and other disorders since the mid-1990's. The image below shows how this magnet is passed across the head [Usually in a figure-8 design]

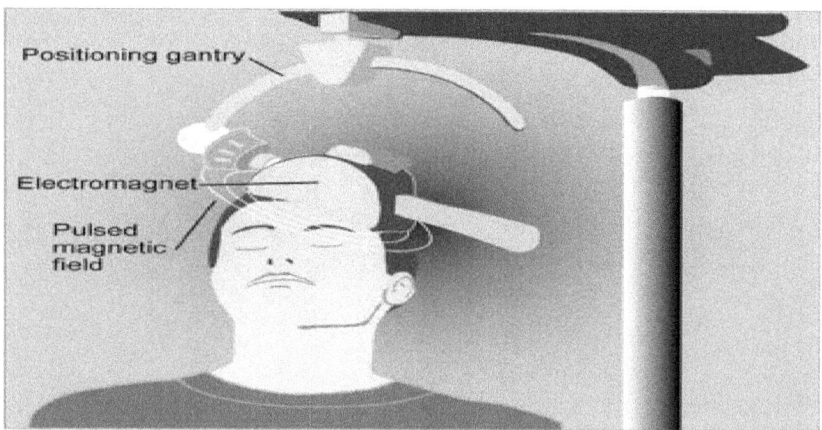

In October 2008, rTMS was approved for use by the FDA as a treatment for major depression for patients who have not responded to at least one antidepressant medication. It is also used in countries such as in Canada and Israel as a treatment for depression for patients who have not responded to medications and who might otherwise be considered for ECT. Unlike ECT, in which electrical stimulation is more generalized and a high voltage is used, rTMS can be targeted to a specific site in the brain. Scientists believe that focusing on a specific spot in the brain reduces the chance for the type of side effects that are associated with ECT. But opinions vary as to what spot is best.

A typical rTMS session lasts 30 to 60 minutes and does not require anesthesia. An electromagnetic coil is held against the forehead near an area of the brain that is thought to be involved in mood regulation. Sometimes the magnet is held in place and short electromagnetic pulses are administered through the coil. The E-M waves easily passes through the skull, and cause stimulation of nerve cells in the targeted brain region. It is believed the E-M field reach down to about 2 inches below the skull. The magnetic field is about the same strength as that of a magnetic resonance imaging (MRI) scan which is a similar E-M invading process that has given us a brand-new perspective in imaging our insides. That brings us to magnetic seizure therapy.

Magnetic Seizure Therapy

While still at relatively low frequencies, The Magnetic seizure therapy (MST) treatments use much higher frequency E-M waves than rTMS uses. MST borrows certain aspects from both ECT and rTMS. Like rTMS, it uses a magnetic pulse instead of electricity to stimulate a precise target in the brain.

Unlike rTMS, MST aims to induce a seizure like ECT, so the pulse is given at a higher frequency than that used in rTMS.

Therefore, like ECT, the patient must be anesthetized and given a muscle relaxant to prevent movement. The goal of MST is to retain the effectiveness of ECT while reducing the cognitive side effects usually associated with it. MST is currently in the early stages of testing, but initial results are promising. Studies on both animals and humans have found that MST produces fewer memory side effects, shorter seizures, and allows for a shorter recovery time than ECT. However, its effect on treatment-resistant depression is not yet established. All these brain-modifying, E-M- field treatments have given way to a new science. From the very slow E-M messaging to the much higher frequency messaging changes things and our study is changed to something called opto-genesis.

Opto-Genetics and Mind Control

While there are many interesting elements of this new science, opto-genetics has two uses we should look at here. The first is to reconstruct an eye for those suffering from blindness. A photo-sensor-array receives the same E-M vibrations of a normal eye and this biologic array has been able to spit out chemically modulated messages similar to an eye and the method is showing signs that will bring sight to the sightless and the brain would still need to learn the chemical messaging and the miracle of light seems to have opportunity. Certainly, miniature CCD cameras are being used to do similar reconstructions as well, but the output messaging is substantially different and training the brain to generate light is difficult.

While that is really useful, we find the most work is done for a more sinister reason as opto-genesis can change what you think or trigger a set of commands learned during training cycles. This neuronal control is achieved using a wide assortment of opto-genetic-actuators like channel-rhodopsin, archaerhodopsin, and many others. The first experiments on rats were not as sophisticated and used an implanted LED emitter that could be pulsed. Today, photo-switches use the secrets of the underwater animal florescence and this can be stimulated through the skull by E-M signals from a phone or other source.

On command the Opto-genetic actuators begin their signaling and true mind control was born. The beginning of this was in the 1990s and was restricted to genetically defined neurons that performed in a spatiotemporal-specific manner by light. In English this was a rudimentary action from a signal. The images below show how direct photonic light emissions were used to modify brain function.

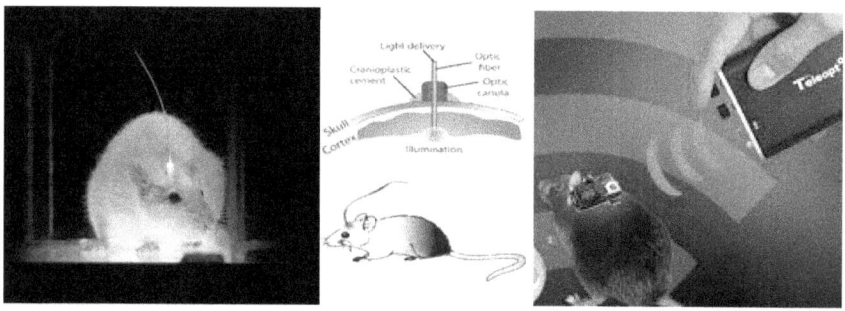

Beginning in 2004, the Kramer and Isacoff groups developed organic photo-switches and scientists were able to modify to alter feeding, locomotion and behavioral resilience in laboratory animals. Soon after, in Frankfurt, they demonstrated that a single gene from the algae *Chlamydomonas* produced large photo-currents and they modified frog brains. By 2005, scientists were controlling behavior of animals and by 2010, opto-genetics was chosen as the "Method of the Year" across all fields of science. It was that earth shattering and still mostly secret. By 2012, Gero Miesenböck optogenetic manipulation neuronal activity to control animal behavior used another biologic called Channelrhodopsin-2 to manufacture blue light messages in rat prelimbic prefrontal cortical neurons. Unfortunately, while all this was going on, Military and government agencies were experimenting on human brain control. In Germany they could turn a group of people hostile to immigrants, into loving acceptors and there are no specifics about what else and who else was being controlled by tiny light pulse messages in the brain as the photo materials could be inserted by injection and training of a 'patient' could be done without him understanding what was going on. With that, I going to leave this section as it makes my heart hurt and visions of the Manchurian candidate keep coming to mind.

Additional E-M Wave Studies

In 1999 scientists began studying how higher frequency E-M field emissions and various visible colors into the cranium could work on rats to "regrow nerves and reduce internal stresses associated with Chronic Stress Disorder". Here are some results.

Growing Back Nerves

Tests are promising and still more work has to be done, however, recent tests had a rat with severed spinal column able to move his legs While there is still a lot of work to do, Continuation of this type of E-M curative response are making researchers very hopeful of the final outcome. Below is a rat outfitted with the normal rTMS device shown to the left.

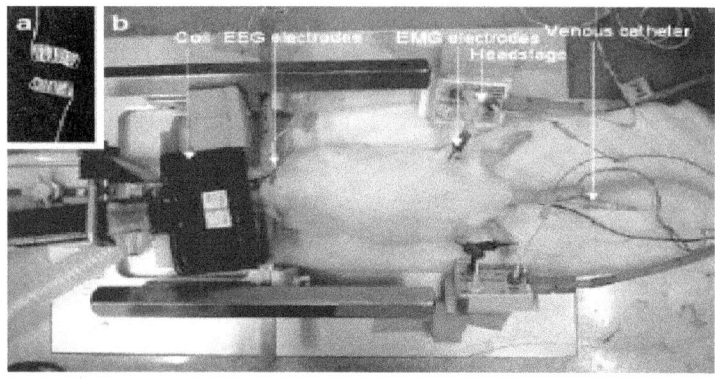

Rodent TMS methodology is applicable to various models of brain injury and to assessment of motor recovery.

Eliminating PTSD

Facilitating fear extinction is clinically important for the treatment of anxiety disorders, such as post-traumatic stress disorder (PTSD). The aim of this next study was to determine if repeated transcranial magnetic stimulation (rTMS) facilitates fear extinction in rats. In this experiment thirty-five rats were conditioned to the fear of a tone by pairing the tone with an electric foot shock Soon there was visible reaction for all subjects, but after fairly high frequency rTMS treatments, those treated lost the aversion to the tone very quickly. This finding suggests that high-frequency rTMS paired with trauma-reminding stimuli enhances fear extinction and that rTMS in conjunction with exposure therapy is potentially useful for facilitating extinction memory in the treatment of PTSD.

Shutting Down the Brain

For this story we go to Cambridge, Massachusetts. A new molecule, along with opto-genetics, has put brain control in the hands of scientists. Researchers from MIT developed a particular protein that is sensitive to red light and enables neurons to be manipulated noninvasively, as the controlling light source is outside the body. They tried green and blue light, but Red penetrated deeper. In addition, this introduced protein allows a large volume of tissue to be influenced simultaneously. Experiments showed that we can, essentially, shut down neural activity in the brains of mice using a light source outside the skull. Currently this is done by injecting a special protein into the cranial area and sticking fiber optic down a hole for introduction of enough light for neuro-silencing, but these new experiments suggest we will no longer have to drill holes. This could lead to more effective treatment of epilepsy and other neurological disorders.

Vision Enhancement

As an offshoot, that Light sensitive protein is also being used to help increase the sensitivity to light of eyes in a somewhat different form of bio-photonic treatments. Some level of vision has even been established. This could lead to more effective treatment of retinitis pigmentosa and other vision disorders.

Brain Scanning

A company named Infrascan makes something called Infrascanner [I don't know where they got the name of their company]. Anyway; it detects the presence of a brain hematoma based on difference in near-infrared light absorption between normal and injured brain tissue. An additional area of research includes detection of oxygen saturation in brain and extremity tissues, edema and concussion to aid assessment and triage of brain-injured personnel on the fly. The success at finding dangerous hematomas in the brain with this light therapy method is astounding. If we modify our doctoring to opto-doctoring, it looks like the death rate of individuals will be reduced, hospital stays will be shorter, insurance rates will go down and our nation will begin to strive.

Diagnostic Monitoring

In diagnostics and functional monitoring, we find near infrared (NIR) diffuse optical spectroscopy. This allows continuous <u>non-invasive monitoring of brain oxygen status in premature babies</u>.

fMRI

Functional magnetic resonance imaging [fMRI] is being expanded using near infrared bio-photonics in a form of opto-genetics that uses gene-based targeting to modulate brain function. I'll bet you are wondering just why that is good. Well it would allow for a minimally invasive method to <u>control Parkinson's disease.</u>

NIR Angiography

In neurosurgery, some biophotonic devices are now in routine use. The new kid on the block is indocyanine green [ICG]-based NIR angiography to find brain issues through the skin. If that doesn't work, fluorescence image guidance is starting to be used for defining the tumor margin in intracranial tumors. All this stuff gets better and better as we may soon have REAL treatments rather than cut out a liver and look for a donor. One thing to look at is <u>killing cells BEFORE messaging creates cancer.</u>

Cell Death

If your cells die, you eventually die. They die all the time and are replaced at a phenomenal rate, but reconstruction requires DNA to send optically coded messages to allow for the construction. Sometimes cell death is not only planned, but important. Cell death is a necessary biological response for the control of multicellular development. Cell death occurs by two principal mechanisms: Programmed Cell Death [PCD] and cell killing by injurious agents.

PCD Death

One might say the destiny of a cell is to die by itself. It is also referred to as "suicide by a cell." A programmed cell death is very orderly <u>and necessary</u> to destroy cells that represent a threat to the organism, such as cells infected with a virus, cells of the immune system, and cells with DNA damage. There are two mechanisms that cause PCD to occur. One is triggered by internal signals from within the cell. An example might be if a protein is damaged in some way the cell will die to insure this does not spread. The other is cell death triggered by external signals where some external damage initiates the cell to die. Cells dying are horrible to watch. First the cell begins to shrink. Then the Mitochondria breaks down making something called cytochrome C. Then the nucleus chromatin degrades and the nucleus turns into little blobs and the DNA and RNA complex cells disintegrate.

DNA

In the early 1980s, a team of scientists demonstrated that the cells of all living beings emit photons at a rate of up to approximately 100 units per second and per square centimeter of surface area and plants seems to generate more. They also showed that DNA was the source of these photon emissions. DNA controls cellular construction so sending out wrong messages can be disastrous.

If the DNA gets hurt and is not destroyed, there can be issues.

What kills DNA?

Deoxyribo-nucleic acid [DNA] is a polymer made up of three major parts.

- Deoxyribose-sugar
- Phosphates
- And Nucleotide sugars [adenine, guanine, thymine, and cytosine]

Yes, people are made out of sugar, but that is not the point here.

Nucleotides connect with each other in these long double helix structures, but some of the unions are not as strong. When Thymine and Thymine connect, it is a weak link and UV light can more easily pull it apart as shown next. Once one of these bonds has separated, the DNA can be easily mutated. We can hope that the cell just dies, but <u>many times it tries to repair itself and we get into trouble.</u>

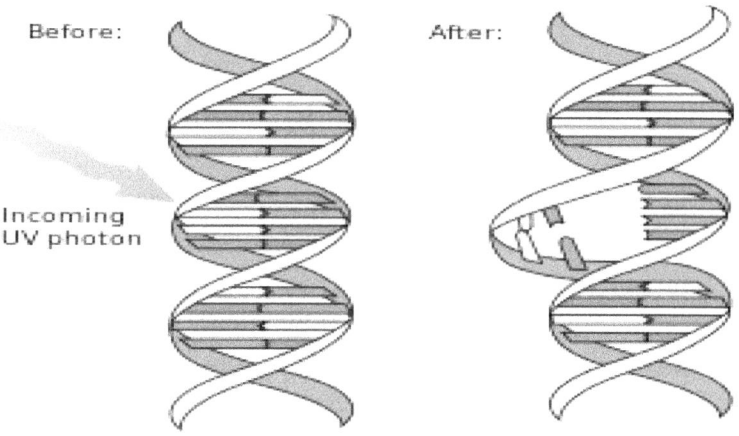

DNA absorbs photons with wavelengths of between 230 and 300nm in the UV range and it is this <u>absorption is mainly responsible for DNA damage, mutation, and death</u>. What we begin to see when out in the sun with 230nm UV hitting us is something we call melanoma as thymine-thymine bonds are broken and the DNA changes what it transmits to other cells. Optical messages ring out and mutations can occur before the DNA finally dies. There are things that can be done.

- <u>Don't let any Thiamin thiamine interfaces in DNA</u>. This might greatly limit functions in people so let's look farther.

- A second thing to do is to <u>eliminate all UV</u>. This is becoming more and more difficult. While I don't go to the beach anymore. This seems like a terrible thing to limit.

- A last thing might be to find out quicker when these DNA breaks occur and <u>kill off the defective Strands</u>. This will take time, but it may eliminate cancers, diabetes, and brain tumors before they even start.

John Hutchison

What if I were to tell you that various microwaves could almost control matter. Certainly, your body is made of matter, so this may be important. For this part of our review, we go to Canada and visit a man named John Hutchison. While not really a bio-photonic researcher, what he does is test what happens with different E-M field s at his home using very powerful E-M transmitters that transmit well outside the visible light spectrum at some type of Microwave frequency. The reason I say "some type" is that he combined many transmitters focused on a single are. The E-M fields combine and we could find frequencies much higher than his initial inputs, but no-one exactly knows those frequencies. This is really bad in that John Hutchison has found things that E-M emissions can do that could harm us. He has been conducting some amazing, well witnessed experiments since 1979 which makes something many call the Hutchison effect. Right now, let me just list the elements known so far. He has demonstrated all of them in the presence of a strange field of electromagnetic waves.

- **Objects** became temporarily invisible
- **Heavy objects** can levitate [even a bowling ball]

- **Things can pass** through each other
- **As they pass** through each other there is no apparent change in either component physical characteristics.
- **Sometimes metals** can become like jelly
- **Sometimes metals melt** without heating

Hopefully your interest has peaked. The focused E-M generators produce "something" and when it is produced, the above things occur to objects in this "Field". Unfortunately, just a tiny change in location or dial position changes the effects.

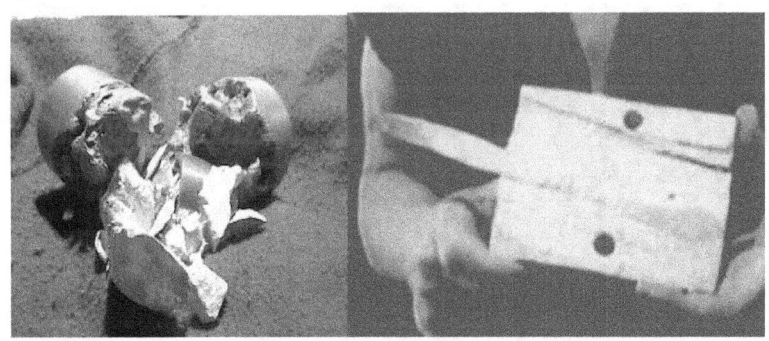

John Hutchison has accidentally found the correct vibrations for particular elements to make them appear invisible to one another so that one can pass through another. The picture above to the right shows how a simple butter knife was pushed through a piece of metal without anyone's help. Now cut in half, the butter knife has become part of the metal. He also has made objects appear to be gravitationally invisible to the earth to allow levitation. During some of his experiments, vibrations mutated the materials to appear to be melted or jelly-like. [See the metal bar above to the left.] Sometimes metals would appear to melt but surrounding wooden objects would not get hot as only the metal structure changed in the field. The effect was as if the objects were changing from this universe to another. The stuff John was finding out was incredible, but someone got scared. In 2006, the Canadian Government went up to John's home and confiscated all of his vibration altering equipment.

While "vibrationally" we may be able to define, modify or even disintegrate a cell, if we are to understand how E-M waves react, we must test the limits and that is exactly where John Hutchison is investigating.

Invisibility and Alchemy

To understand a little more about making cells disappear or changing dangerous cancer into something benign, it may be interesting to examine what has been done in the past with high voltage E-M fields as characterized in previous experiments. While there is no public ascertain of true successes, we can gain information from partial successes. The first to review has been called the Philadelphia Experiment that was done in Philadelphia of all places.

Philadelphia Experiment-Like John Hutchison's experimentation they were able to make things disappear and reappear, and make objects go through other objects and make things levitate, but in this experiment, they added living tissue in the form of sailors. While much of the experimentation was never divulged, what we find is that even the sailors became invisible enough to be "embedded" into the. Those that were not killed or embedded went mad as the brain cells were scrambled.

Most of the reports of that experiment simply can't be verified bot one thing that keeps coming up is that the ship holding the E-M generators disappeared and reappearing at a different location hundreds of miles away in an instant. Rather than suppressing the experiment limited successes, it should be heralded as modification of cellular structure might holds a key to treatments and E-M fields hold the key. Just to complete this modification of cell with E-M field section, let me quickly bring up what you could call modern alchemy.

Modern Alchemy- To build up large E-M fields, various techniques have been employed but not to modify cells. Instead we are turning Lead into Gold. I know alchemy is a bad word and instills an image of sorcery, but in the Atomic Age, it is almost commonplace to transmutate elements into other elements. The following list describes the successes that have been reported. Today most are done with the "Atom Smashers" where magnets as long as towns are used build fields of unbelievable strength so using these techniques might not be useful when treating people, but it does show a direction that we might go to modify cells by some miniature rotating magnetic field or something. I made a short list of atomic structure modifications to finish off this whole concept.

Date	Researcher	Method	Initial Mat'l	#	End	#
1920s	Franz Tausend	A	Mercury	80	Gold	79
1923	A. Miethe	B	Mercury	80	Gold	79
1924	Hantaro Nagaoka	B	Mercury	80	Gold	79
1924	Smits & Karssen	B	Lead	82	Mercury	80
1927	Walter Russell	B	Oxygen	8	Nitrogen	7
1935	Lord Rutherford	C	Nitrogen	7	Oxygen	8
1936	Various	C	Platinum	78	Gold	79
1938	Hahn & Strassman	C	Uranium	92	Ba + Kr	56+36
1939	Various	C	Thorium	90	Radium	88
1960s	Jnana & Caro	A	Lead	82	Gold	79
1972	Soviet Physicists	C	Lead	82	Gold	79
1980	Glenn Seaborg,	C	Lead	82	Gold	79
1986	Various	C	Mercury	80	Gold	79

By the way; the **A**-means Harmonic Alchemy [not really frequency based]—**B**-means High voltage/high frequency distillate—**C**-means Nuclear Accelerator Bombardment. Notice that the most converted element is Gold. I guess there is a flare for sorcery in our modern-day scientists.

I know I've gone way outside the comfort zone of some who were just wondering about what color light would cure erectile dysfunction, but if just one of these ideas sparks a new thought in the treatments of injury, diseases, defect, and enhancement of people, animals and plants I think it has been worth the trouble. With that, let's go over some of the things that were addressed in this book and see if you got the basis of details from my explanations. First, I redefined light.

Redefinition of Light

I have been using photons, light, and E-M fields interchangeably during this book, but there is a huge distinction. It might be useful for me to address this difference so less confusion might be had. Unfortunately, the dictionary provides us NO HELP at all. Here is what it says.

> *Light is E-M radiation that is visible, perceivable by the normal human eye as colors between red and violet, having frequencies between 400 terahertz and 790 terahertz and wavelengths between 750 nanometers and 380 nanometers.*

This makes no sense. If a blind person sees "light" in a dream or thought, is it light? ----Of course, it is, in fact, all light is made by the brain not by the eyes. As one gets near the speed of light perception of colors are substantially different than when one is standing still so velocity counters any normal definition.

Let me just say while photons are truly Electro- magnetic waves photons are NOT light at all. It is a processed thing derived by whatever activates rods and cones to cause some response. This presumably could be accomplished by electromagnetic pulse, some type of chemical reaction, or other phenomenon. Instead of the eye, many of the treatments and focus in this book has been DNA perception and transmission of E-M fields for communication, repair, diagnostics, update, and transfer. While U-V wavelengths were the major emphasis because of the type of tools we have today. We may find other more useful frequencies that could help us as well.

E-M Field- Electromagnetic radiation of any frequency or wavelength. Of course, this includes the more mundane "visible light" wavelengths, x- rays, cosmic rays, radio waves, the wavelengths that are so slow we can't transmit them through air, Ultraviolets, and the oddball long infrared and microwave frequencies.

This is a more complete definition and the one I used in this book. You won't always be able to find devices that output some of these wavelengths directly definition.

Light Perception

While trying to define light is almost impossible I think there are some definitions we can establish. First of all, does everyone see "red" the same way? I'm sure you have asked this question. If light is simply an interpretation by the brain of chemical exchanges made by the bio-photonic exciting of rod and cones in the eye there can be little thought that everyone sees the world the same. One might think my red looks blue to another. I'm not talking about color-blind people here; I'm talking about normal eyesight interpretation by cells in the brain. But maybe this is a fallacy.

Since the science of Anthropics came along, more and more now believe everyone sees things the same. In fact, everything is regulated by people seeing, touching and interacting with them. As an example, when Albert Einstein was asked the simple question--- If a tree falls in the woods and no one is around, does it make a sound? ------His answer was simple and complex at the same time.

He said, "There is no forest and there is no tree."

Light is the same thing if there is no one to interpret photonic action, there is NO LIGHT. Light does not exist, but photons and E-M waves do exist in a Space and Time constant viewpoint. I hope that clears up things for you.

A second question might be, "Do photons exist?" The easy answer is they don't exist as something you can feel [most of the time] Some knuckle-head might say, "We should never use light for these experiments as it doesn't exist and using photons seems to be problematic with their halfway existing."

I could go faster into Anthropic science here as is greatly affects how we interpret all of this and what it all means, but it gets a little bizarre and I think you have had enough bizarre already.

Conclusions

Bio-photonics is such a broad topic, it's hard to know where to begin, but it seems to be the most important leap in therapy of all sorts of nasty diseases.

Blood circulation and Diabetes- Seems like cells want to rejuvenate themselves but they can't remember how. Blasting them with <u>red makes them remember</u>. Diabetics love it. <u>Infrared lasers do similar tasks and blood flows</u>. We found that <u>blood has photo-receptors or eyes</u> and sending the right frequency to them relaxed the otherwise constricted veins choking off blood flow.

Heart-Brain- Hopefully you have a better appreciation on how one might use the E-M interaction of a heart-brain to cure disease. Still a lot of work is needed in this field as every day a new possibility arises. The idea that the heart could be a communication channel relay between the head-brain and the body, may enable new treatments for nerve damage.

Cancer- What's not done to destroy cancer? Proteins injected and irradiate making them send out bio-photonic messages that help kill cancer while pinpointing them for a doctor's own blaster. Put some mistletoe nearby and it sends out bio-photonic messages that end up destroying the mass. With new experimental E-M fields that completely change matter or even make it invisible may introduce more treatment methods.

Brains- You name it in the area of bio-photonics and the brain is sampled. They track calcium, track messages, look for hematoma, and put parts of the brain to sleep all with light. New Infratonic emissions now allow for extremely low frequency introduction which seems to modify "thought". Added to a high energy magnetic source and relief of many symptoms are truly changing how we repair the brain.

Erectile Dysfunction- There is no need for Viagra or even something to set the mood. Once processed, a simple blue light does the trick and rigidity is back in play.

Fluorescence- Cells in some species commonly make visible light. The cuttlefish is a master and hypnotizes its prey by flashing colors and sequences by simply regulating bio-photonic emissions in its skin cells. Applications of fluorescence to test for cancer and other defects is still another exciting avenue for advancing photonic medicine.

Pineal Gland- With cells similar to cones and rods of the eye, this thing uses light to regulate sleeping and sexual understanding. It's a shame it's in the center of the brain and it's a shame they still force fluorine into the water of children that have not reached puberty so that sexual confusion is amplified.

Plants- emit coded optical message to scream for help and send messages that have nearby plants protect themselves. Sometime fungus is used as a plant's fingers. If you want bio-photonic giant plants eat them after just being picked.

Cooking pulls the life out of them and their photonic emissions used for treatments in cancer are completely eliminated.

Eggs- When they want the other eggs to die----bio-photonic messages are sent. If they want the other eggs to catch up so all will hatch at the same time, a different message is sent. It's all about timing and E-M messaging.

Faith Healing- There seems to be a similarity between Buddhist, CHI, Hypnotherapist, and faith healing methods that are associated with placing hands near the body as if the messaging between the healer and the patient is a weak single like the bio-photonic emission registered by Kulian and sensitive photometric systems. The success rates indicate this messaging is powerful and not well understood.

Halo- While bio-photonic emissions are usually weak, something can cause the halo to grow as was noted in Moses and others from the Bible history.

Light- I briefly went over how light doesn't exist, but instead is "Manufactured" in the brain.

Anthropic Science- While briefly discussing how there is a controlling function in our "reality" that forces a level of order, I did not get into so much detail simply because it would confuse things even more.

In the Beginning- I tried to open a new vision about how God created this unbelievable reality for us and how light and life were so tightly connected. Apparently, Moses knew a lot way back when he wrote Genesis. We think we understand so much more than those ancient people but concepts presented in the Biblical history are <u>only now</u> becoming understandable to us.

We know very little about the secrets of bio-photonics, but every year more and more discoveries are being made and it is an exciting time. While cancer deaths are still going up at an alarming rate, I think we may have turned the corner and will soon be saving more and having fewer people die in hospitals in agony and suffering when just a little light could save them. Fewer people will have legs removed as circulation is halted by diabetes and brain dysfunctions will start to be controlled. Photons are not light, but all E-M waves should be reviewed for how they might help our bodies.

Thanks for reading.

The End

About the Author

Steve Preston is a long lime author of scientific, esoteric facts. His books focus on the painful truths rather than whitewashed details that make us comfortable. If you are interested in the truth instead of comfort, please review other works by Mr. Preston as shown in the following list. The images are some from Egypt taking the older version of taxi. To the right the writer is shown in the Jewish Negev desert of Israel where the Dead Sea Scrolls were found. I made these travels so you wouldn't have to.

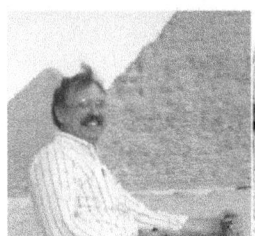 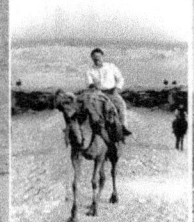 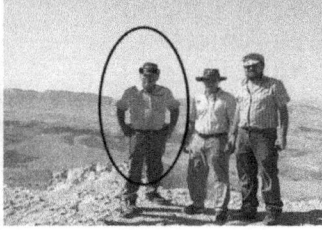 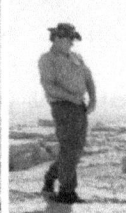

To the left below are a couple of pictures as we searched the New Zealand caves possibly visited by the ancient Maori and the last image is of the author investigating the statues on the Acropolis in Athens Greece. Luckily, light was everywhere I looked.

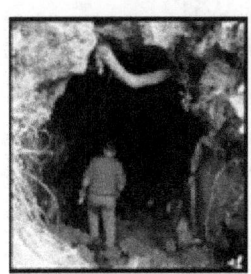 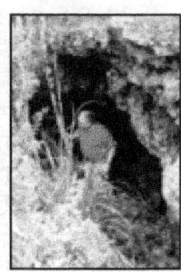 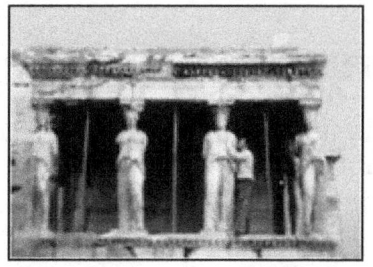

History of Mankind Series
20th Century To The End Of Time
The Second Creation of Man
The Creation of Adam and Eve
A New View of Modern History
Close Look at Ancient History
The Antediluvian War Years
The First Creation of Man
Man After The Flood

Modern American Topics
History of Powerful Women
Promote the General Welfare
Modern Misconceptions
Our Very Odd Presidents
American School Disaster
The Bad Side of Lincoln
Can We Save America?
Great American Quiz
Humans on Display
Consensus Science
Monsters are Alive
US History Errors

Prehistoric America
Who Discovered the Americas?
Mysterious PreIncan Journey
Phoenicia and the Lost Jews
Romans found America

Prehistoric Technology
Amazing Technology
Mysterious Pyramids
Incredible Titans
Anakim Gods

Prehistoric History
Creation and Death of Dinosaurs
Kingdoms Before the Flood
When Giants Ruled the Earth
Not from Space

Reality Science Anomaly
Our 12-Dimensional Universe
Mystery of Photons and Light
Meaning of Life and Light
Incredible Nikola Tesla
Is Time Travel Possible?
Biophotonics and Healing
Vibrational Matter
Slip Through a Wall
Anthropic Reality

Historical Fiction
Conrad and the Flood
Secrets of Washington
Shama and the Tower
Naille and the Exodus
Religious Anomalies

Biblical History
Does Science Confirm the Bible?
History Confirmed By The Bible
Abraham to Moses
Adam to Abraham
Adam's First Wife
Moses to Jesus

Moses Studies
Moses Story Part 1
Moses Story Part 2
Expanded Genesis
Exploring Exodus
Exploring Genesis

Christian Studies
Differences in the King James Bible
Why the King James Bible Failed
Understand the New Testament
Old Testament Used By Jesus
New Testament Mysteries
Allah' God of the Moon
Errors in Understanding
Old Testament Mysteries
New look at the Bible
Incarnations of God

Biologic Anomaly
Tracing Cro-Magnon to Jesus
God Didn't Make The Ape
DNA of Our Ancestors
Homo Erectus as a Man
DNA Anomalies
Races of Men
Lizard People

Wars
America's Civil War Lie
Behind the Tower of Babel
World War with Heaven
Four Armageddons
World War Before
World War Zero
Six Deaths of Man
Driven Underground

Egyptian Studies
Truth About Hyksos Pharaohs
Scythians Conquered Ireland
Mysteries of the Exodus
Egyptian Foreigners
Moses Saved Egypt
Secrets of Thoth

Metaphysic Science Anomalies
Releasing Your Consciousness

Understand your Heart
Vampires among Us
Awaken the Departed
Self, Soul, Spirit
Life Resonance
 Self-Virtualization
Of Heaven and Hell
True Happiness

Flight & Space Travel
Ancient History of Flying
Anomalies in Flight
Living on Venus
Space Anomalies
Where UFOs Go
Martians

Angels and Demons
Sex Crazed Angels
The Antichrist
The Devil